WAVERLY HILLS SANATORIUM

A HISTORY

LYNN POHL

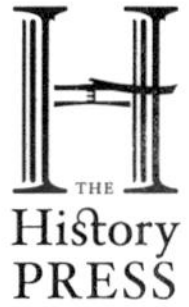

Published by The History Press
Charleston, SC
www.historypress.com

Front cover: Main sanatorium at Waverly Hills. *Caufield and Shook Collection, 76039, Archives and Special Collections, University of Louisville.*

First published 2022

Manufactured in the United States

ISBN 9781467149990

Library of Congress Control Number: 2022933361

To Kevin, Ezra, Helena, Chi, Millie, and Russel
There are no other three people and no other three cats I would rather be quarantined with.

CONTENTS

ACKNOWLEDGEMENTS

My deep dive into the history of Waverly Hills Sanatorium began with the support of coworkers at the Filson Historical Society: Heather Potter invited me to look at Edward Arthur's photographs in early 2019, and Jennie Cole, Abby Glogower, and Patrick Lewis gave me the opportunity to give a talk and write an article about the Filson's records relating to tuberculosis and Waverly Hills. I am deeply grateful to Peggy Moran and Don Moran, who gave me constant encouragement and provided valuable feedback on an early version of the manuscript. Emma Johansen shared her father's story with me, and her father let me include it in this book.

Staff at archives in Louisville generously responded to my questions and requests, pulled materials for me to look at, and sent me scans and files. Special thanks go to Mary K. Marlatt at University of Louisville Kornhauser Health Sciences Library and Carrie Daniels, Tom Owen, Elizabeth Reilly, Kyna Herzinger, and Cassidy Meurer at the University of Louisville Archives and Special Collections. Amanda Clark at the Louisville Metro Department of Public Health and Wellness gave me the opportunity to look through the Board of Health minutes, and Scott Utterback sent me a selection of *Courier-Journal* images. Thank you to the Filson Historical Society, the University of Louisville Archives and Special Collections, and Kornhauser Health Sciences Library for the use of images from their collections.

I am very thankful for the many people who talked with me about the history of Waverly Hills Sanatorium and read what I had written. Dr. Morris

Weiss Jr. did both, and I have been fortunate to learn about important parts of Louisville's medical history from him. I am especially indebted to Jody Caldwell, who took the time to critique several drafts of the manuscript, offering extensive advice and pointing out needed corrections every time. He and Jeremy Songer were part of numerous conversations about Waverly Hills. Kristin Regala, Teresa Hines, and Erica Coulter read versions of my manuscript and made much-appreciated comments and suggestions. Teresa Hines also shared her family's story with me, as did other people by email. John Amerine shared his and his wife's research with me.

An immense amount of my free time at home during 2021 was spent researching and writing. Much love and appreciation to my husband, Kevin Smith, and our teenage children, Ezra and Helena, for enduring the ups and downs of my full immersion into this project and for being my favorite people.

While I had the luxury of laboring at a computer, all kinds of workers on the front lines of the pandemic were trying to safely do their jobs and provide necessary care and services to others. They merit far more than my gratitude.

INTRODUCTION

High on a hill on the south side of Louisville in Jefferson County, Kentucky, stands a four-story stone and brick Tudor Gothic Revival building with a partial fifth floor and tower. Completed in 1926, the building is the only major surviving structure of Waverly Hills Sanatorium, a sprawling complex providing treatment for tuberculosis patients from 1910 until 1961. After serving as a residential facility for the aging from 1962 to 1981, the property passed through the hands of several owners. For almost two decades now, the current incarnation of Waverly Hills Sanatorium has offered public tours and paranormal investigations.[1]

On a beautiful sunny afternoon in April 2019, my teenage son and I joined a group tour of the sanatorium building. The tour guide led us through multiple sections of the building, including the long sun porches and patient rooms, an operating room, and the rooftop with grand views of the surrounding area. I was grateful for the opportunity to walk through such a massive physical artifact of Waverly Hills Sanatorium and to see up close the spaces that defined the experiences of so many patients and employees. Despite the deterioration and emptiness of the building, it was not difficult to imagine the porches and rooms filled with patients reading, gossiping, playing cards, enduring boredom and their symptoms, and worrying about their future and loved ones back home. It was not difficult to imagine the orderlies, nurses, physicians, and other staff moving about those spaces doing their jobs, providing care, and navigating their own relationships and problems.

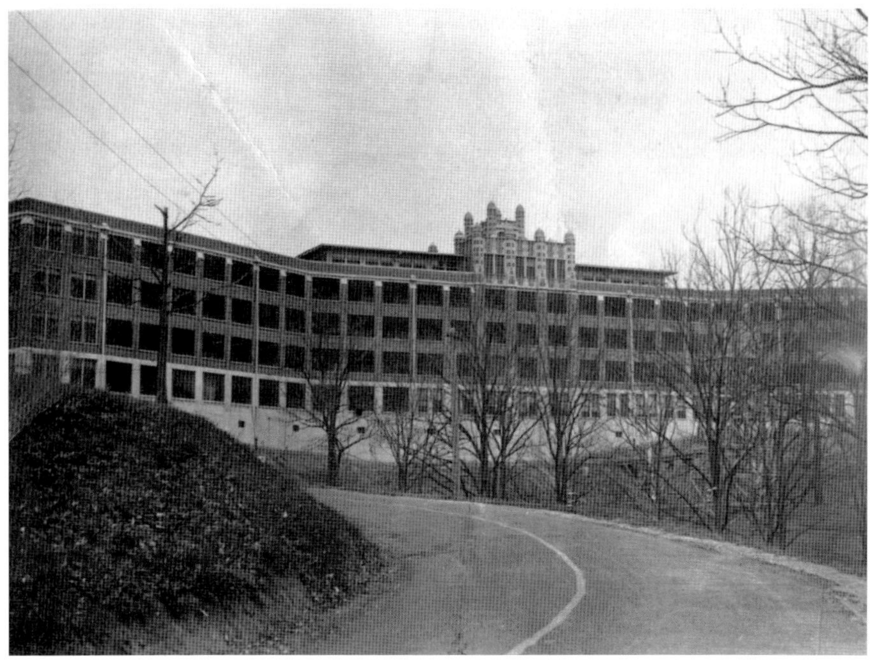

The back side of the main sanatorium building at Waverly Hills, circa 1926. *Edward Arthur Waverly Hills Photograph Collection, 019PC9.20, Filson Historical Society.*

My interest in touring the colossal structure, and afterward in writing this history of Waverly Hills Sanatorium, stemmed in part from my work as a medical historian. In past years, I had researched and taught about the early twentieth-century history of tuberculosis, the public health campaigns that tried to prevent its spread, and the mix of desperation and hope that drove many patients to seek sanatorium treatment. When I taught classes on the history of health and medicine at Louisville's Spalding University, my students and I wondered why there was so little documented history written about Waverly Hills Sanatorium.

In early 2019, the donation of a remarkable set of photographs to Louisville's Filson Historical Society, where I work, prompted me to book the tour at Waverly Hills Sanatorium and to investigate its history more deeply. The photographs had belonged to Edward A. Arthur, who was diagnosed with tuberculosis in the 1910s and lived at Waverly Hills in the 1920s. He worked as treasurer and then as business manager at the sanatorium, possibly after he had been admitted or partly recovered as a patient. He met and married Rosa Ann Williams (called Anna), and they had two children: their son Edward was born in 1926 and their daughter

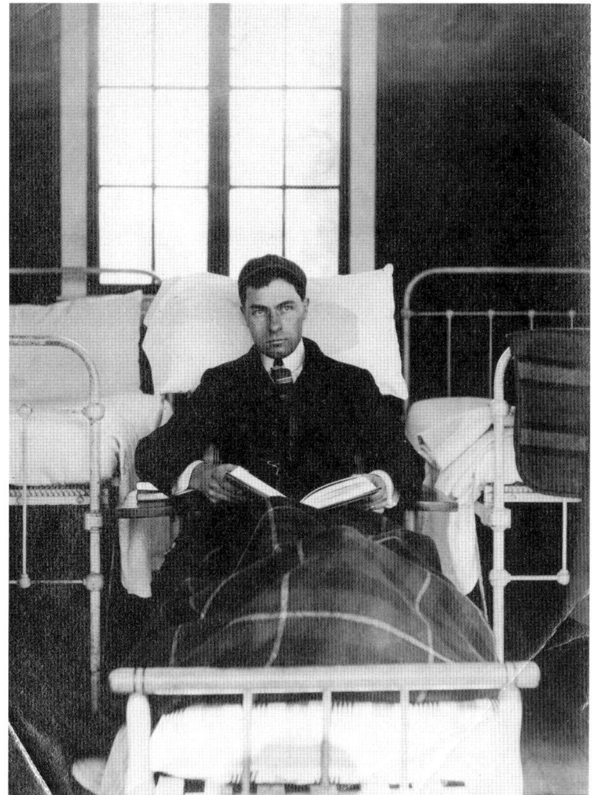

Right: Edward Arthur posing in a suit in bed at Waverly Hills, circa 1920s. *Edward Arthur Waverly Hills Photograph Collection, 019PC9.13, Filson Historical Society.*

Below: Edward Arthur with his family at Waverly Hills, circa 1928. *Edward Arthur Waverly Hills Photograph Collection, 019PC9.22, Filson Historical Society.*

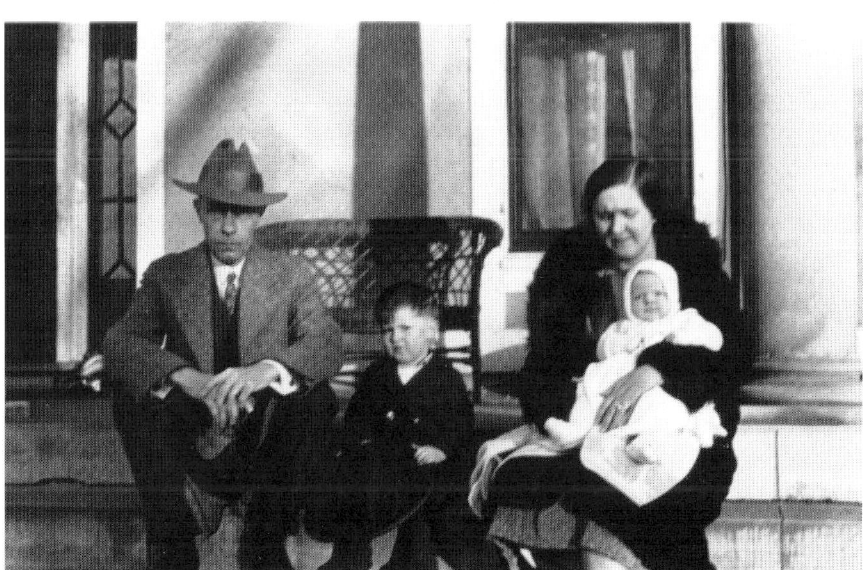

Catherine in 1928. On June 29, 1929, the forty-nine-year-old Edward Arthur died at Waverly Hills of pulmonary tuberculosis and possible complications of myocarditis.[2]

Most of the photographs of Waverly Hills left behind by Edward Arthur date from before the 1926 opening of the sanatorium building still standing today, and many appear throughout the first half of this book. They provide a glimpse of the social relations forged at Waverly Hills, depicting employees and patients posing in front of the Waverly Hills administrative building and pavilions that opened in 1910 and the children's pavilion that opened in 1916. They also present more somber views of the effects of tuberculosis, including photographs of a physically frail female patient.

As I began to research the history of Waverly Hills Sanatorium, wanting to discover more about the buildings and the people in the photographs, I did not expect to find much. Many of the institution's records were destroyed during the Ohio River flood of 1937 when they were stored in downtown Louisville, and others were destroyed after the sanatorium closed in 1961.[3] As a result, there appear to be few surviving patient records or administrative files. Over time, however, I found that a range of existing records—including newspaper articles, published reports, letters, personal recollections, and Board of Health meeting minutes—offered surprisingly rich documentation.

Among the local records documenting the history of Waverly Hills is a series of digitized issues of the *Louisville Leader*, a Black-owned newspaper that ran from 1917 to 1950.[4] A number of *Louisville Leader* articles referred to Esther Maxwell Barrens, who worked at Waverly Hills from 1926 until her death in 1954. Born in Tennessee in 1882, Esther Maxwell moved to Louisville in 1907, married Charles Barrens in 1908, and sometime later adopted her daughter Marie Barrens.[5] In the summer of 1926, she became the first Black nurse hired at Waverly Hills. Before this point, Black patients admitted to Waverly Hills were housed in segregated wards of the hospital that opened in 1913 to treat advanced cases of tuberculosis. In 1926, the new sanatorium building opened to white patients only, and the administration used the hospital for advanced cases to create a separate division at Waverly Hills for Black patients. The division was staffed by Black physicians and nurses at a time when no other public medical institution in Kentucky offered positions to Black professionals. At the same time, the Black hospital's overcrowded facilities stood in stark contrast to the new sanatorium for white patients. Esther Barrens was sometimes the only nurse on staff in the Black hospital. Yet she took on additional responsibilities, arranging informal

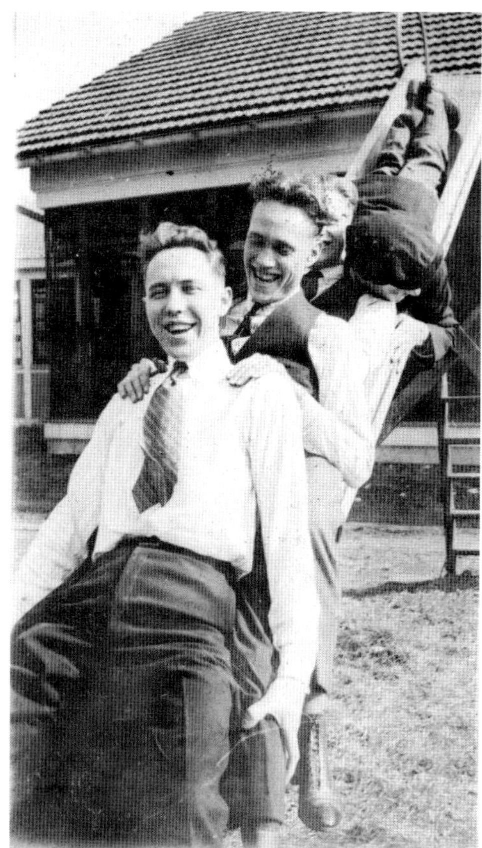

Right: Young men at Waverly Hills Sanatorium, circa 1920s. *Edward Arthur Waverly Hills Photograph Collection, 019PC9.26, Filson Historical Society.*

Below: Young women at Waverly Hills Sanatorium, circa 1920s. *Edward Arthur Waverly Hills Photograph Collection, 019PC9.26, Filson Historical Society.*

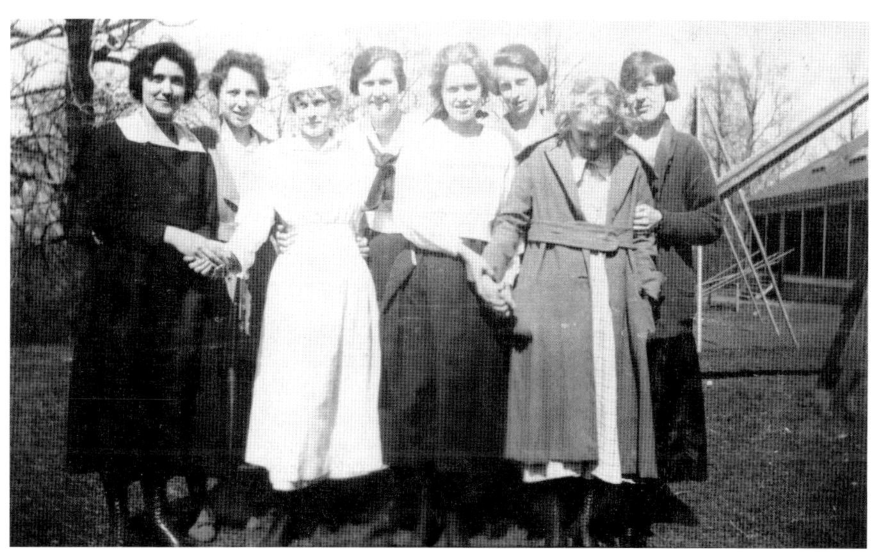

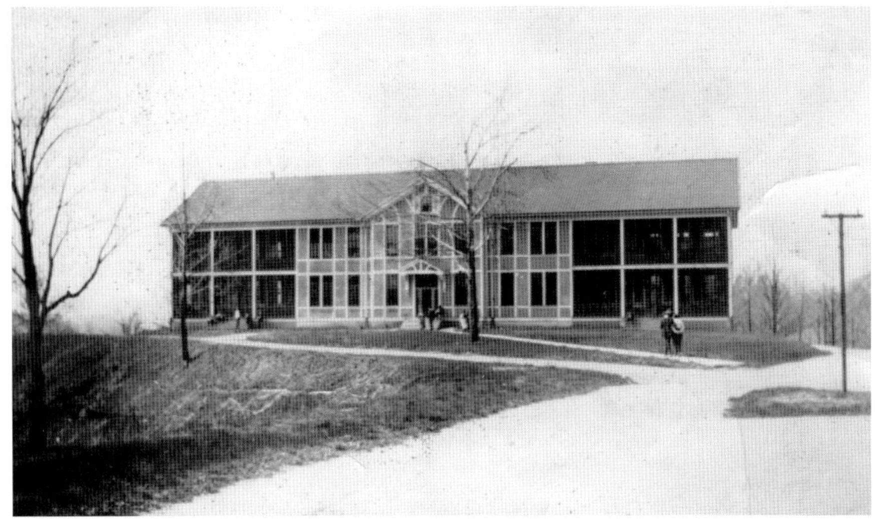

The hospital for advanced cases at Waverly Hills that became the Black hospital in 1926. *Edward Arthur Waverly Hills Photograph Collection, 019PC9.26, Filson Historical Society.*

elementary school classes for children at the Black hospital and serving as a liaison between the hospital and local Black associations.

Edward Arthur and Esther Barrens are two of the tens of thousands of patients and employees who lived and worked at Waverly Hills during its half century of history, and they may have never crossed paths in the few years their time at the institution overlapped. This book aims to tell the history of the many people and many parts of Waverly Hills Sanatorium. Individual patients and employees had very different experiences at Waverly Hills, depending on their race, their age, their stage of illness, their job, their years of treatment or employment, the buildings where they lived or worked, the friends they made there, and their connections to people outside the sanatorium. Yet across time and in disparate spaces, patients and staff members like Edward Arthur and Esther Barrens contributed to a shared aim and a collective story, as they tried to salvage health and make lives for themselves within the confines of Waverly Hills, in the face of one of history's most debilitating and deadly diseases.

AUTHOR'S NOTES

NOTE ON NAMES OF ORGANIZATIONS

Different organizations and entities contributed to the founding of Waverly Hills Sanatorium and its management over the years. Here are the most important ones:

Kentucky Anti-Tuberculosis Association. This private organization was formed by a group of Louisville men and women in 1905. It was renamed the *Louisville Anti-Tuberculosis Association* in 1909 and the *Louisville Tuberculosis Association* in the early 1920s.

Board of Tuberculosis Hospital. The Kentucky Anti-Tuberculosis Association put a bill before the Kentucky state legislature in 1906 creating the Board of Tuberculosis Hospital and authorizing city and county tax levies for the establishment and maintenance of a public tuberculosis institution. The Board of Tuberculosis Hospital oversaw the institution that opened as Waverly Hills Sanatorium from 1910 until 1942.

Louisville–Jefferson County Board of Health. This public entity was established in 1942, with the merger of the Louisville Department of Health and the Jefferson County Board of Health. Upon its creation, the Board of Health took over management of Waverly Hills Sanatorium from the Board of Tuberculosis Hospital.

NOTE ON SPELLING OF WAVERLY HILLS SANATORIUM

Several variations of the spelling of Waverly Hills Sanatorium were used from before its opening until long after its closing. Variations include *Waverley Hill*, *Waverley Hills*, and *Waverly Hills*. *Sanatorium* was sometimes spelled *sanitarium*, a nineteenth-century term for a health resort or institution for the treatment of a variety of "nervous" or chronic diseases. *Sanatorium* was generally the term used for an institution for the treatment of tuberculosis. For consistency, except in quotations or when discussing the purchase of the Waverley Hill estate in 1908, this book uses the spelling *Waverly Hills Sanatorium* and the shorthand version *Waverly Hills*.

NOTE ON NAMES OF WAVERLY HILLS SANATORIUM BUILDINGS

Waverly Hills Sanatorium included many different buildings over time. Here are what the main ones are called in this book:

Main administrative building. The main administration building was one of the original structures of Waverly Hills Sanatorium that opened in 1910. It included the laboratory, staff offices, dining areas for patients and employees, and staff quarters. It was incorporated into the design of the new sanatorium building that opened in 1926.

Women's pavilion, *men's pavilion*, and *children's pavilion*. The men's and women's pavilions opened in 1910 and were located on each side of the main administration building. The children's pavilion opened in 1916 and was located next to the women's pavilion. These pavilions housed white patients. They made up what was called the *sanatorium* in Waverly Hills reports from the 1910s, a term that also encompassed nearby cottages and tents—some of which may have housed Black patients. The children's and women's pavilions were incorporated into the design of the new sanatorium building that opened in 1926, and the men's pavilion was moved and used as quarters for male employees.

Hospital for advanced cases. The hospital opened in 1913 and included racially segregated wards for the treatment of white and Black patients with advanced cases of tuberculosis until 1926. Black children were housed in the hospital with Black adult patients.

Main sanatorium. This is the building still standing today. It was constructed between 1924 and 1926 and connected to the original main administrative

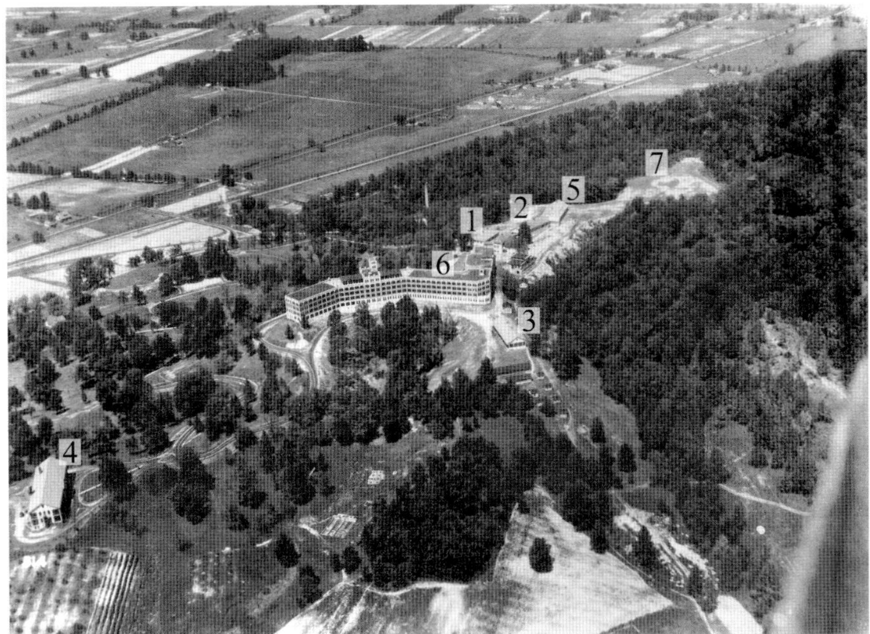

Aerial view of Waverly Hills, circa 1926. Herald-Post, *94.18 0757, Archives and Special Collections, University of Louisville.*

The buildings labeled with numbers are:
(1) Main administration building, opened in 1910
(2) Women's pavilion, opened in 1910
(3) Men's pavilion, opened in 1910 and moved in 1924
(4) Hospital for advanced cases, opened in 1913 and became the Black hospital in 1926
(5) Children's pavilion, opened in 1916
(6) Main sanatorium, opened in 1926
(7) Site of the nurses' home, opened in 1929

building and women's and children's pavilions. It housed only white patients for all but the last few years of its existence as a tuberculosis sanatorium, and it is typically referred to as the "main sanatorium" in administrative records.

Black hospital. When the main sanatorium opened to white patients in 1926, the hospital for advanced cases was converted into a hospital for Black patients only. Another facility for Black patients opened in 1933, and an addition was made in 1943. These buildings were usually referred to as the "Negro division" or "Negro hospital" in administrative records and newspaper accounts. This book refers to these facilities as the Black hospital.

Chapter 1

"A LINGERING DISEASE"

Tuberculosis is one of the oldest infectious diseases known to civilization. Pulmonary tuberculosis, affecting the lungs, is the most prevalent form of the disease, but tuberculosis bacteria can also invade and affect other parts of the body such as the bones, the lymph nodes, and the brain. In the lungs, the bacteria are usually contained by specialized cells of the immune system in a hardened nodule and remain a latent, noncontagious infection, causing no symptoms. In about 5 to 10 percent of people who are infected, however, the bacteria slowly multiply and develop into an active case of tuberculosis, with symptoms gradually worsening over time. These individuals' breathing, coughing, sneezing, and spitting can infect others in close contact who inhale airborne particles carrying tuberculosis bacteria.[6]

Before 1882, when the specific bacterium that causes tuberculosis was identified, relatively few people suspected tuberculosis was an infectious disease. The disease was most commonly called *consumption*, a term first used in Europe in the 1300s to describe illness involving the respiratory system and causing dramatic weight loss over time. The name evoked a body consumed by disease, wasting away over time. Use of the term *consumption* persisted into the twentieth century, usually interchangeably with the term *tuberculosis*, though sometimes with its own meaning. A *Louisville Courier-Journal* article from 1915 explained to its readers, "Tuberculosis is the beginning stage, consumption is the awful ending."[7]

The term *tuberculosis* was coined in the early 1800s and derived from the Latin word *tuber*, meaning root or swelling and referring to the growth of nodules in the tissue of the lungs. While physicians, like their patients, continued to use the more popular term *consumption* through the 1800s, many noted their observations of tubercles—masses of tissue, blood, and phlegm coughed up by patients. In the 1830s and 1840s, Dr. William McDowell of Louisville described these tubercles as ranging from "the size of wheat grain to that of a pea." Dr. McDowell wrote of examining the lungs of patients, listening for crackles and other sounds of a diseased lung. Physicians also used percussion, tapping their fingers on each side of the patient's chest and back to see if they could hear a dull resonance indicating a mass or consolidation in the lungs or a cavity formed from tissue destroyed during the progression of the disease.[8]

Certain symptoms of consumption were readily discernible by ordinary people as well as by physicians. In the early stage, a patient might have a dry cough or pains in the chest—symptoms common to many other diseases and thus difficult to diagnose. Kentuckians wrote about more advanced stages of consumption in vivid terms, describing "drenching night sweats," constant coughing, "spitting blood," lack of appetite, weakness, weight loss, and "a hectic fever." The final stages of tuberculosis were often marked by sunken cheeks and hollow eyes, swollen extremities, diarrhea, and a respiratory rattle (also known as the "death rattle"). A terrifying hemorrhaging from the nose and mouth—the result of ruptured blood vessels in the wall of a tuberculous cavity—could cause patients to drown in their own blood.[9]

Tuberculosis was a leading cause of death in the nineteenth century, when the disease was associated as much with the wealthy as with laborers and immigrants. Historians often note how the consumptive look—pale and emaciated, with flushed cheeks—became fashionable among authors and artists. Most people writing about the disease, however, did not romanticize its devastating effects on the body. A diagnosis of consumption heralded a less certain future and the possibility of an early and painful death. In 1873, Agatha Logan of Lexington, Kentucky, wrote matter-of-factly about her recent diagnosis of consumption: "Dr Bush made an examination of my lungs and told me they were very seriously involved—a fact I have known all along—of course I am in no immediate danger for consumption is a lingering disease but I have no hope or expectation of ever being well again." Logan aptly characterized consumption as a "lingering disease," one in which symptoms could come and go and progress slowly over years. She married Louis Marshall two years after her diagnosis and lived another thirty-one years. Others suffered through a quick decline. In 1850, James Stewart of Wolf Lake, Indiana, described

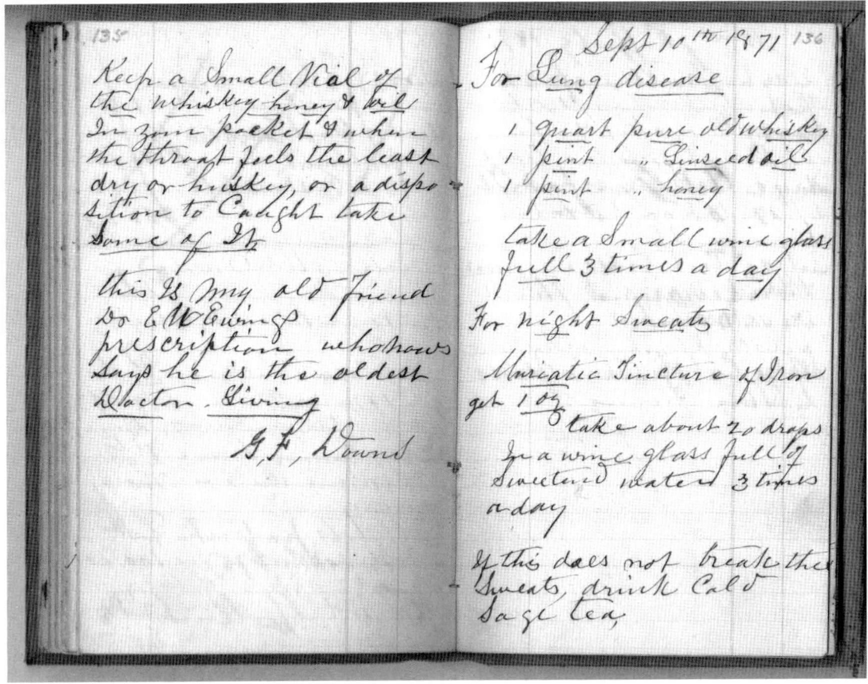
135

Keep a Small Vial of
the whiskey honey & oil
In your pocket & when
the throat feels the least
dry or huskey, or a disposition to Caught take
Some of It

this Is my old friend
Dr E McEwings
prescription who now
Says he is the oldest
Doctor Living

G.F, Downs

Sept 10th 1871 136

For Lung disease

1 quart pure old whiskey
1 pint " Linseed oil
1 pint " honey

take a Small wine glass
full 3 times a day

For night Sweats

Muriatic Tincture of Iron
get 1 oz
take about 20 drops
In a wine glass full of
Sweetend water 3 times
a day

If this does not break the
Sweats, drink Cold
Sage tea

Kentuckians often relied on home remedies, such as this recipe from 1871 of "pure old whiskey," linseed oil, and honey for "lung diseases." *George F. Downs memorandum book, John Harding papers, folder 101, Mss. A H263, Filson Historical Society.*

a friend's death from consumption after spending most of the nine-month duration of the disease limited to his bed. "He suffered the most exquisite pain while confined," Stewart wrote, "but death has finally closed the door. He suffered without murmuring, he repined not, he fell asleep as we hope in the arms of his savior."[10]

Treatments for consumption in the nineteenth century drew on long-held beliefs in the value of fresh air, a suitable diet, and gentle exercise, at least for those not forced to do hard labor. People suffering from consumption usually remained at home. Most hospitals at this time were public or small charitable institutions serving low-income patients who did not have family members to care for them or who could not afford to call a physician to their home.[11]

Patients with the monetary means to do so sometimes sought treatment by taking sea voyages or traveling to the Northeast, to the West, or—for a few years in the early 1840s—to Kentucky's Mammoth Cave. Louisville's Dr. John Croghan, who bought Mammoth Cave in 1839, spearheaded the creation of an underground village for "invalids" and "consumptives." One of Dr. Croghan's patients, Oliver Hazard Perry Anderson, wrote several letters documenting his time living underground. In a letter dated December 12, 1842, a few months after Anderson took up residence in his underground "cottage," he wrote of the cool air in the cave as "very tonic and fine for exercising, manifestly imparting strength; its humidity is fine for the lungs." He also complained about the smoke from fellow residents' stoves aggravating his cough. No one in the cave had "grown better," he wrote, but the residents agreed "they would be worse out and hence contentment generally pervades our little community."[12] He departed the cave in January 1843 after two of the occupants died and four others had left, noting, "I don't look as well as when I entered the cave."[13] While the cave village was short-lived and of doubtful therapeutic value, at its best it provided a place for the inhabitants to keep one another company and to expose themselves to the cave's steadily cool temperatures.

Widespread belief in the restorative value of certain types of air, such as the bracing climate of the mountains, fed into the sanatorium movement

6. In. the. Mammoth. Cave. Edmondson. Co. Ky. Sept. 9-11-1932
Margaret. Schafer. at. the. first. consumptive. house

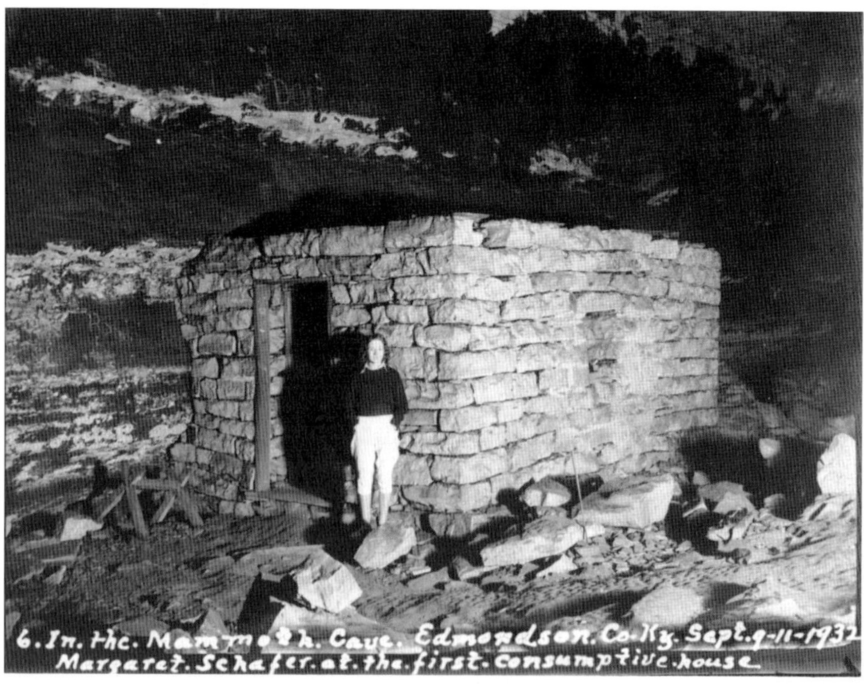

Remains of a "consumptive house" at Mammoth Cave. *Rogers Clark Ballard Thruston Photograph Collection—Kentucky Counties, TC-1101, Filson Historical Society.*

that began in the late nineteenth century. In 1884, Dr. Edward Trudeau opened one of the first sanatoriums for the treatment of tuberculosis in the United States, the Adirondack Cottage Sanatorium at Saranac Lake in New York. The main therapeutic aim of a tuberculosis sanatorium was to admit patients in the early stages of tuberculosis and then build up their bodies' abilities to overcome the disease and regain their health—all in a regulated institutional setting. Kentuckian William L. Allen's letters recorded his experiences as a patient at Trudeau's sanatorium in the early 1900s. He noted, "I am outdoors all the time, save that devoted to meals," and he described his current setup: "I am lying on my piazza-bed reading the book of Job, my individual spit box on one side, a box of cough drops and an atomizer also within easy reach." He wrote, "The diet is a trifle monotonous and put together too much with the idea of nutrition and not enough with the idea of novelty of taste." He also complained about the tedium of bed rest: "Here I am, feeling all right—as if I could walk ten miles—yet kept flat on my back all day, and allowed no excitement. As long as I have any temperature." Like other patients enduring the symptoms of tuberculosis, he expressed his dim hopes for a full recovery, writing that he was "peeping into a rather dubious future."[14]

The establishment of sanatoriums for the treatment of tuberculosis converged with the spread of new understandings of microscopic germs as the cause of certain diseases. In 1882, German physician Robert Koch identified the bacterium causing tuberculosis and called it *Tubercle bacillus*, which was often shortened to "TB" and later renamed *Mycobacterium tuberculosis*. Before this point, tuberculosis was generally thought to be a hereditary disease, not a contagious one like smallpox. Moving forward, physicians and public health officials could more reliably diagnose tuberculosis through laboratory analysis of a person's sputum (a coughed-up mix of saliva and mucus) and, later in the twentieth century, with X-rays and skin tests. They learned how tuberculosis was an airborne disease transmitted through an infected person's coughing, spitting, or sneezing, especially in prolonged contact with others in unsanitary and unventilated environments. With this knowledge, public health officials focused on measures to try to eradicate sources of contagion, identify cases of tuberculosis, and prevent the spread of the disease.[15]

Proponents and proprietors of tuberculosis sanatoriums argued that institutional treatment served both a preventative and a curative function by isolating tuberculosis patients from the public and giving them the opportunity to recover from their disease. Their efforts won widespread

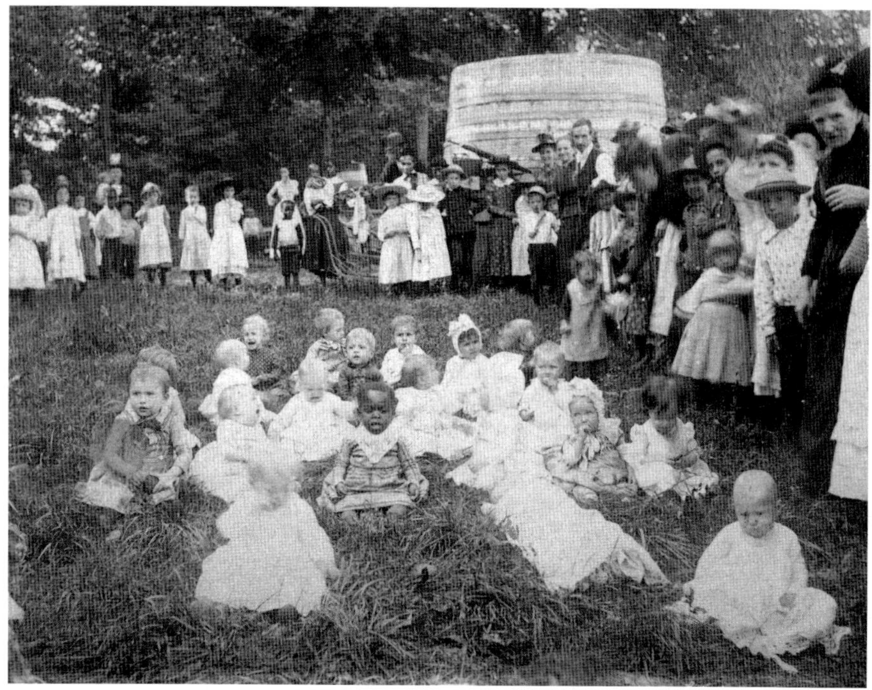

These Louisville children and adults took part in a steamboat "fresh air excursion" in the summer of 1892. The label on the back advertises, "Boats loaded with sick. Doctors, medicines, medicated foods, car fare, and conveyances free for the needy sick." *HEA-4, Filson Historical Society.*

support as tuberculosis persisted as a leading cause of death into the early twentieth century. The number of tuberculosis sanatoriums in the United States increased rapidly from 34 with 4,485 beds in 1900 to 536 with 673,338 beds in 1925, and they included not just private institutions like Trudeau's but also publicly funded ones like Waverly Hills Sanatorium.[16]

Chapter 2

LOUISVILLE'S ANTI-TUBERCULOSIS CRUSADE

Founded in 1778 as a shipping port along the Falls of the Ohio River, Louisville became the largest city in Kentucky by 1830. The city's economy diversified after the Civil War with the expansion of railroads and manufacturing, and the population quadrupled from fewer than 50,000 in 1850 to over 200,000 in 1900. At this beginning point of the twentieth century, African Americans made up 19 percent and immigrants 10 percent of the city's residents.[17]

Louisville's rapid population growth contributed to problems of overcrowded housing and the spread of infectious diseases. In the early 1900s, health officials reported that tuberculosis ranked as the number-one cause of death and accounted for approximately one out of seven deaths in the city. An estimated two to three cases were contracted every day, and as many as five hundred city residents died from the disease every year. According to the head officer of the city health department, Dr. M.K. Allen, the high rates were particularly troubling because tuberculosis was "perfectly preventable."[18]

Louisville's crusade against tuberculosis began in earnest in May 1904, when Dr. Dunning S. Wilson published an editorial in the *Louisville Times* calling for the formation of a tuberculosis association and the establishment of tuberculosis sanatoriums. One of the first physicians to respond to the plea for action was Dr. Jacob A. Flexner. He and Dr. Wilson gained the support of Eleanor Tarrant, director of the Neighborhood House, which provided social and educational services to Louisville's immigrants and low-income residents. Other social reformers and men and women of wealth and political prominence joined the cause, leading to the incorporation of the Kentucky Anti-Tuberculosis Association in June 1905.[19] The association published its aims in a report on its first annual meeting in early 1906:

> *First: To educate our people as to the nature of the disease; the method of its communication; the safeguards to be used to prevent its spread; and its curability in our home, as well as other climates, if treated in time by modern methods.*
>
> *Second: To erect and maintain Sanatoria for the accommodation and treatment of patients afflicted with the disease.*
>
> *Third: To provide treatment at their homes for such as cannot be accommodated in Sanatoria.*[20]

The Kentucky Anti-Tuberculosis Association, which changed its name to the Louisville Anti-Tuberculosis Association in 1909 and the Louisville Tuberculosis Association in the early 1920s, operated as a privately funded organization. In addition to securing large donations from wealthy benefactors, the association embraced a new form of fundraising involving the broad solicitation of small donations. In 1908, it joined one of the first annual nationwide Christmas seal campaigns, selling seals to the public for a penny apiece to be attached to the envelopes of holiday mail. The seals helped to spread awareness about tuberculosis and to fund anti-tuberculosis programs. On May 17, 1909, the association held its first "ten-cent campaign," with volunteers going door to door to request a donation of a dime from each family or household. The Colored Women's Improvement Club took charge of collecting dimes from Black residents in 1911.[21]

The first public program of the Kentucky Anti-Tuberculosis Association brought Dr. S.A. Knopf, a tuberculosis specialist who helped found the National Association for the Study and Prevention of Tuberculosis in 1904, to speak at Louisville's Warren Memorial Presbyterian Church. After the talk on December 11, 1905, the Kentucky Anti-Tuberculosis Association distributed free copies of Dr. Knopf's essay, "Tuberculosis as a Disease of the Masses and How to Combat It." In future years, the association's educational campaign made use of speeches, newspaper articles, placards, school programs, state fair booths, radio recordings, and films.[22]

"CONSUMPTION GOES ABOUT LIKE A DRAGON SPITTING DEATH"

Louisville's anti-tuberculosis crusade involved not just the Kentucky Anti-Tuberculosis Association but also many other private organizations and municipal agencies. Their efforts epitomized the variety of reforms associated with the Progressive Era in the early twentieth century. Like reformers across the country, anti-tuberculosis leaders in Louisville spearheaded educational campaigns, lobbied for the passage and enforcement of legislation, and provided services to those in need—all with the aim of addressing some of the worst effects of rapid urban growth and industrialization. In this work, they targeted the "laboring masses" who had become associated with tuberculosis by the 1900s.[23]

An important aim of public health advocates was to teach about germs and contagion, which were still new concepts to many people in the early twentieth century. Their main message emphasized both the dangers and the preventability of germ transmission. They explained how tuberculosis bacilli spread in invisible and insidious ways, while also arguing that careful actions on the part of individuals could prevent the transmission of germs. The disease was not just a "medical problem" for physicians to address but also a "social condition" requiring sanitary management and "the attention and assistance of every man and woman."[24]

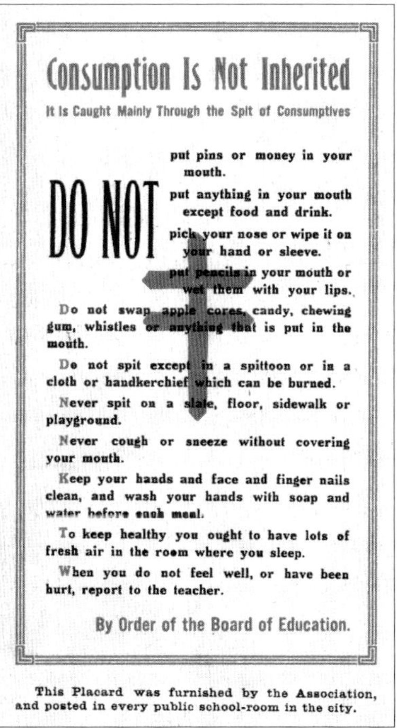

Educational campaigns taught that tuberculosis was an infectious disease and its spread could be prevented through these kinds of health habits. Six Years' Work, *1911, vol. 4, Louisville Tuberculosis Association Minutes, Mss. BA L888a, Filson Historical Society.*

One of Louisville's most active anti-tuberculosis leaders was Temple Bodley, a lawyer who was diagnosed with the disease in 1903 at the age of fifty. He recovered and lived another thirty-seven years. From 1905 to 1907, he gave a series of speeches educating the public about tuberculosis and lobbying for a publicly funded sanatorium. Like other public health advocates, Bodley spoke of the dangers of tuberculosis germs lurking everywhere, as the bacilli lodged in the lungs and were expelled through an infected individual's coughing and spitting: "It has been calculated that a single consumptive has, in a single day, coughed up from his lung and expectorated four thousand millions of these living germs." The germs in dried-up sputum, he asserted, could survive for months and even years in dark or dry conditions, to be sent airborne as dust at a later time by a broom or a gust of wind.[25] Bodley spoke of this threat in ominous terms:

> *In nearly every community—in this community—consumption goes about like a dragon spitting death. It has been doing so for centuries....It invades alike the houses of the poor and the rich....No man, no woman, no child is safe from it. In Louisville one out of every seven person you meet will presumably die of it. The poison is in the streets, in the public buildings, in private houses, in the air.*[26]

As Bodley lectured to middle-class men and women and business leaders, he highlighted the economic and social repercussions of tuberculosis. The disease was "most fatal at the very time when the lives of its victims are of the greatest economic value to the community, between the ages of 16 and 45." The money lost to tuberculosis, he argued, "would build a Panama Canal or make a million dollar endowment every year for each of a hundred universities, hospitals and other public benefactions." Only California had higher death rates from tuberculosis than Kentucky and Tennessee, and most of those who died from the disease in California had traveled there for treatment. The high death rates in Kentucky, he said, were due to "ignorance of the disease and our carelessness." In 1905, Bodley warned members of the Louisville Women's City Club that their class and racial privileges would not serve as sure protection from the disease. "Over ten per cent of all deaths among the leading white races are due to Tuberculosis," he said, referencing the belief of many middle-class white Americans that they made up the "leading" segments of society.[27]

Anti-tuberculosis leaders encouraged the public to follow modern tenets of healthful living: washing their hands before meals, eating green vegetables, getting a good night's rest, sleeping with the windows open, and making annual visits to a physician "no matter how well you feel." Those who developed "a habitual cough and expectoration" were told to go to their physician or a tuberculosis clinic to have a microscopical examination of their sputum.[28]

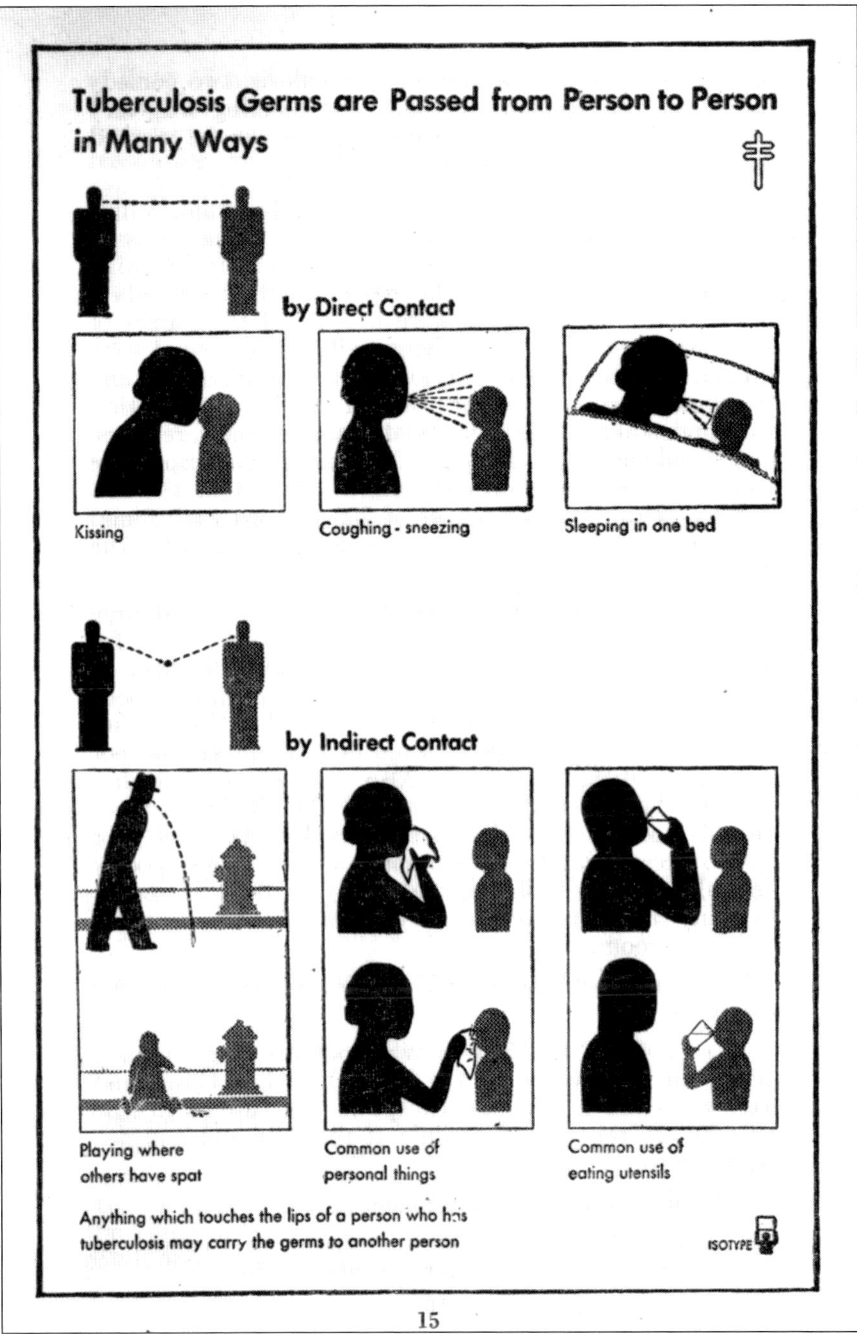

Educational campaigns taught how tuberculosis could spread from person to person. 34th Annual Report of the Louisville Tuberculosis Association, *1938, pamphlet 614.542 L888, Filson Historical Society.*

Individuals diagnosed with tuberculosis were advised to take numerous precautions to avoid spreading the disease to others. Dr. M.K. Allen instructed tuberculosis patients to avoid spitting anywhere except in a cup, ideally one filled with a disinfectant solution of water and carbolic acid. They should empty the cup twice a day and clean it thoroughly with more carbolic acid solution and then with boiling water. When away from home, patients should spit into handkerchiefs or pieces of cloth to be boiled in water or burned. "The kissing of consumptive patients," Dr. Allen warned, "is extremely dangerous." Their bedroom should be "large, airy and well lighted" and frequently disinfected. He directed male patients to be clean shaven and keep their hair short, due to the belief that such styles were more hygienic than beards and long hair. All patients, he advised, should seek out sun and fresh air.[29]

Following these recommendations was a near-impossible feat for the many urban dwellers who lived with family members in crowded housing conditions, struggled to afford basic necessities, and lacked ready access to private physicians. One way the Louisville municipal government tried to encourage personal cleanliness was to provide public bathhouses where "clean towels, soap, and a bath are furnished free." In 1911, there were two public bathhouses for white residents and one for Black residents. Charitable associations also offered some basic services. The Babies' Milk Fund Association provided supplies of milk to the children of low-income families. Inspections of dairies helped to ensure the milk was not from tubercular cows, which could transmit *Mycobacterium bovis*, another bacterial cause of tuberculosis.[30]

Legislation offered another weapon against tuberculosis. Beginning in 1902, the city required physicians and public health officials to report cases of tuberculosis, and in 1905, the city enacted an anti-spitting ordinance authorizing arrests and fines for offenders. Spitting was targeted both as a widespread habit among men, including those who chewed tobacco, and as an involuntary symptom of tuberculosis patients. The aim was to prevent spitting on the surfaces of sidewalks, streetcars, and other public spaces and to encourage spitting into cups instead. In 1911, the city health department solicited local newspapers for help publicizing how "careless spitting" passed germs from the sick to the well. It printed 100,000 placards to be distributed on streetcars and by policemen to "working men leaving factories." The health department claimed success with this campaign, announcing that "education did the work with less than a hundred arrests." Yet health officials continued to complain for decades about "promiscuous spitting."[31]

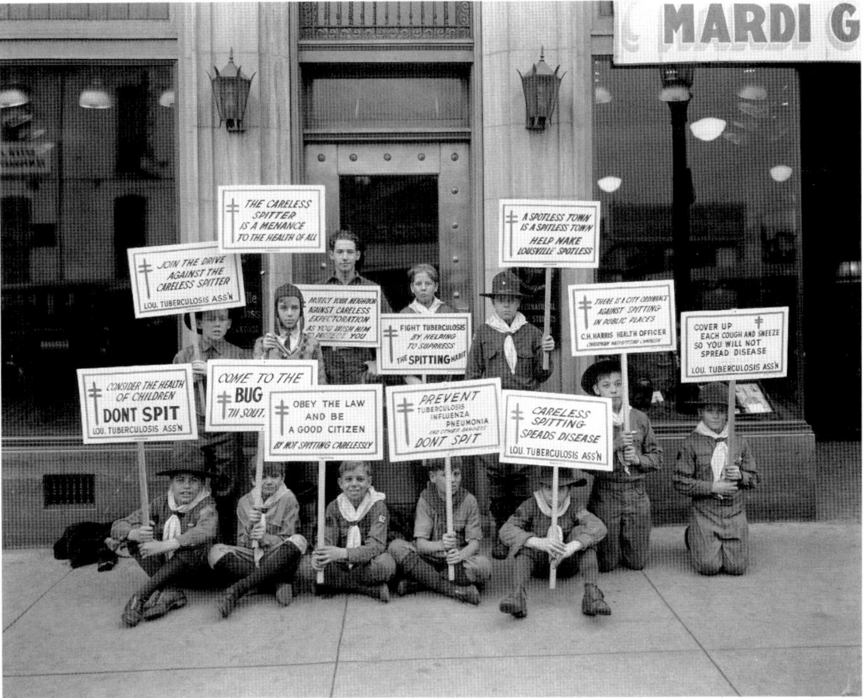

MARDI G
THE CARELESS SPITTER IS A MENANCE TO THE HEALTH OF ALL
JOIN THE DRIVE AGAINST THE CARELESS SPITTER
LOU. TUBERCULOSIS ASS'N
AGAINST CARELESS EXPECTORATION
FIGHT TUBERCULOSIS BY HELPING TO SUPRRESS THE SPITTING HABIT
A SPOTLESS TOWN IS A SPITLESS TOWN
HELP MAKE LOUSVILLE SPOTLESS
THERE IS A CITY ORDINANCE AGAINST SPITTING IN PUBLIC PLACES
C.H. HARRIS HEALTH OFFICER
COVER UP EACH COUGH AND SNEEZE SO YOU WILL NOT SPREAD DISEASE
LOU. TUBERCULOSIS ASS'N
CONSIDER THE HEALTH OF CHILDREN
DONT SPIT
LOU. TUBERCULOSIS ASS'N
COME TO THE
BUG
OBEY THE LAW AND BE A GOOD CITIZEN
BY NOT SPITTING CARELESSLY
PREVENT
TUBERCULOSIS
INFLUENZA
PNEUMONIA
DONT SPIT
CARELESS SPITTING SPEADS DISEASE
LOU. TUBERCULOSIS ASS'N
Boy Scouts' anti-spitting campaign, 1928. *Caufield and Shook Collection, 096674, Archives and Special Collections, University of Louisville.*

While many of Louisville's anti-tuberculosis campaigns targeted the "laboring classes" in general, white officials often singled out Black workers in particular. In the early 1900s, Dr. M.K. Allen pointed to domestic laborers as a serious threat to the health of white families: "In this city, where much of the domestic help is colored, is it not perfectly possible that families are endangered to a great degree from this fact?" Like many other white officials and physicians, he repeated racist rhetoric blaming the "habits" and "environments" of African Americans, and he failed to acknowledge the vast system of racial discrimination and exclusion severely restricting educational, employment, and housing options for Black Louisvillians.[32]

Decades later, a 1924 survey of health care in Louisville echoed stereotypes about the "susceptibility" of certain racial and ethnic groups to tuberculosis: "Negroes and persons of German and Irish stock, which races suffer in this country from a special susceptibility to disease of the lungs and particularly tuberculosis, are sufficiently numerous to influence unfavorably the general death rate and sick rate of the city." While blaming these groups of Louisvillians for the city's high rates of tuberculosis, the survey also documented the dilapidated condition of the city's tenements—buildings rented out as multifamily dwellings to many low-income, Black, and immigrant residents. Louisville's tenement housing, according to the study, typically had little ventilation, no indoor plumbing or water supply, and outdoor privies. The two inspectors within the newly created tenement house division of the local health department were stretched thin in their work enforcing sanitary standards of the city's housing ordinance. Landlords were not compelled to improve the construction and plumbing of tenement housing, and renters had few options to move elsewhere.[33]

The Louisville Women's City Club, consisting primarily of white middle-class women, involved themselves in anti-tuberculosis efforts on several fronts. Members drew attention to housing problems, citing their survey of Metropolitical Life Insurance records in 1924 to underscore that "the highest death rate is where the poorest housing is found....The densest area is found from Broadway north to the river and from Campbell west to 15th street." They mentioned the work of the Louisville Tuberculosis Association and the Louisville Urban League in helping to fumigate and clean up property where someone had died from tuberculosis.[34]

Women's City Club members met with health officials to discuss the possibility of establishing clinics in industrial workplaces and sending domestic laborers to those clinics. They proposed issuing certificates to those who were examined and shown to be free from tuberculosis, "as an aid to the patient and a protection to those associated with them." They suggested that "on account of the fear generally felt by most people at the word 'tuberculosis,' the clinics be known as general health clinics and not specifically for tuberculosis." A local physician asked for the help of the Women's City Club legislative committee in lobbying for a law "compelling the examination of employees at restaurants, soda fountains, domestic servants, etc. and making it necessary for them to obtain a certificate of health."[35] Public health advocates saw this focus on identification of tuberculosis cases as part of the broader effort to prevent the disease from spreading. Clearly, however, the spread of tuberculosis they were most concerned about was to middle-class families who went to restaurants and soda fountains and hired domestic laborers.

ESTABLISHING THE BOARD OF TUBERCULOSIS HOSPITAL, A FREE DISPENSARY, AND HAZELWOOD SANATORIUM

The creation of an institutional infrastructure in Louisville and Jefferson County to diagnose and treat tuberculosis began in the first decade of the twentieth century, when the Kentucky Anti-Tuberculosis Association helped to establish a free tuberculosis dispensary and two sanatoriums. In 1906, the association put a bill before the state legislature creating the Board of Tuberculosis Hospital and approving Louisville and Jefferson County tax levies to fund a public sanatorium—the institution that would open as Waverly Hills Sanatorium four years later. The bill was passed and signed into law in March. Once the members of the Board of Tuberculosis Hospital were appointed to a term of four years by Louisville mayor Paul C. Barth, they began to lobby the city and the county to increase their tax levies for the sanatorium. Funds from the taxes were allowed to accumulate while the board searched for a location for the sanatorium and planned its design.[36]

As the Board of Tuberculosis Hospital worked on funding and plans for the public sanatorium, the Kentucky Anti-Tuberculosis Association turned its attention to opening a dispensary (a free public clinic) for tuberculosis

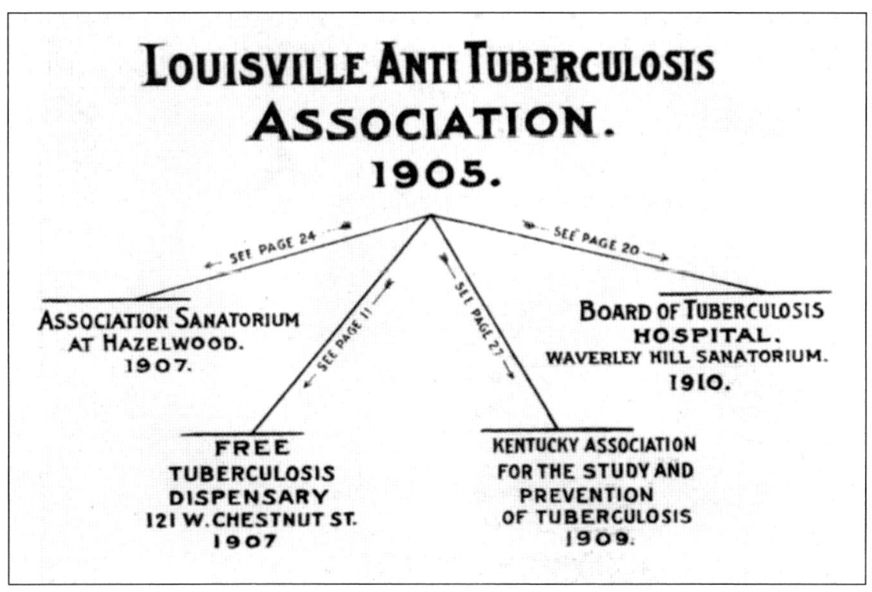

Louisville Anti-Tuberculosis Association chart showing the organizations and institutions it helped to establish. Six Years' Work, *1911, vol. 4, Louisville Tuberculosis Association Minutes, Mss. BA L888a, Filson Historical Society.*

patients in 1907. Charles Goldsmith, chair of the association's dispensary committee and one of the founders of Louisville's Jewish Hospital, led this process through the opposition of residents downtown. The association first signed a lease for the dispensary at 208 West Chestnut Street, but resistance from neighbors to a tuberculosis clinic so close to their homes convinced the landlord to refuse possession of the building. The association then signed a lease for another location at 121 West Chestnut Street and moved equipment into the building in the middle of the night, before the neighbors realized what was happening. According to a history of Waverly Hills, "Many attempts were made to dislodge the dispensary" before nearby residents begrudgingly accepted it.[37]

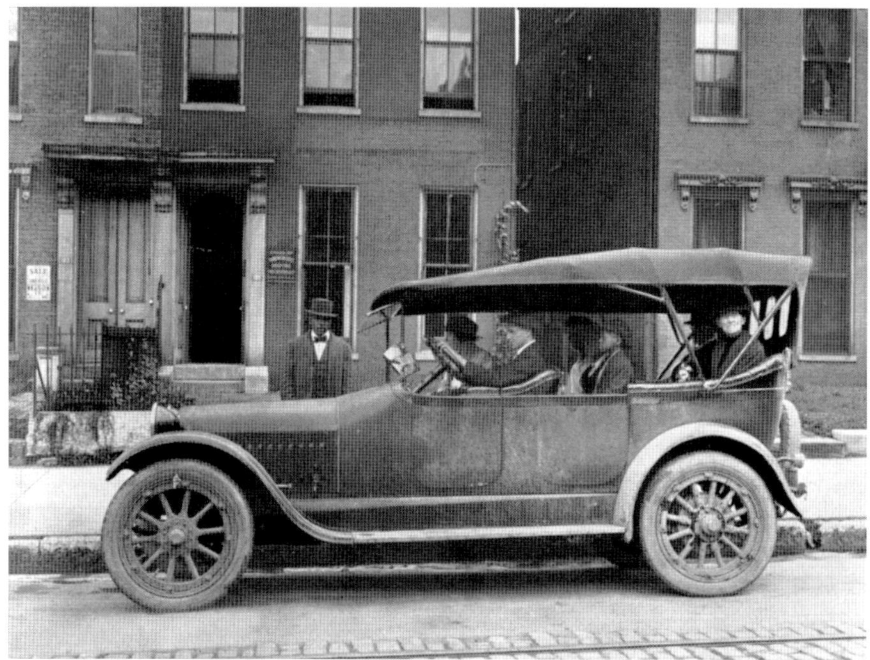

Above: White and Black passengers in a car at the Free Tuberculosis Dispensary at 121 West Chestnut Street. Report of the Board of Tuberculosis Hospital, *rare pamphlet 362.16 B662 1916, Filson Historical Society.*

Opposite, top: White and Black patients waiting to be examined at the Free Tuberculosis Dispensary. Few medical offices or hospitals were racially integrated in Louisville until the 1950s and 1960s. Report of the Board of Tuberculosis Hospital, *rare pamphlet 362.16 B662 1916, Filson Historical Society.*

Opposite, bottom: A physician examining a young patient at the Free Tuberculosis Dispensary. Report of the Board of Tuberculosis Hospital, *rare pamphlet 362.16 B662 1916, Filson Historical Society.*

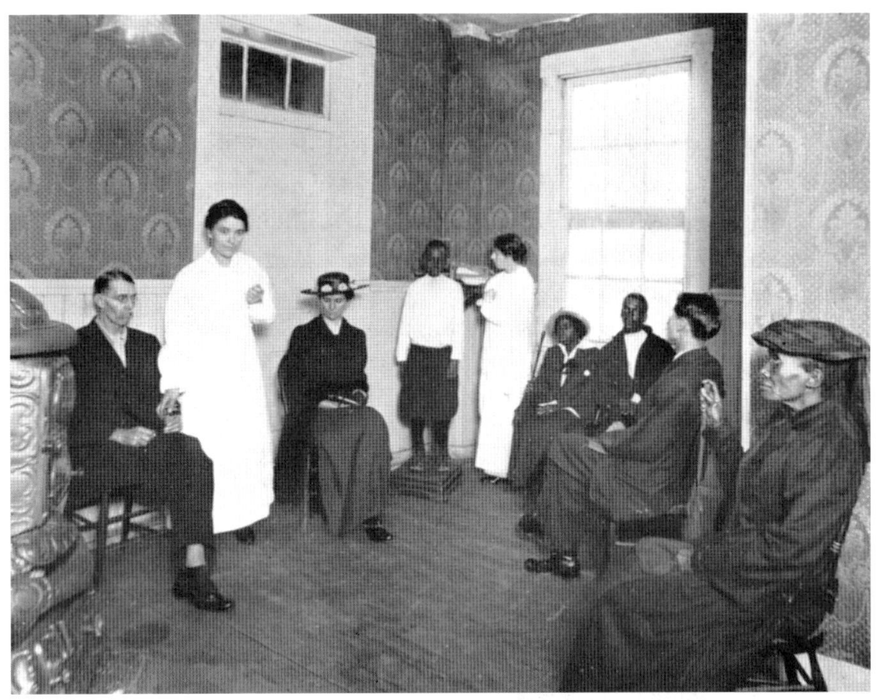

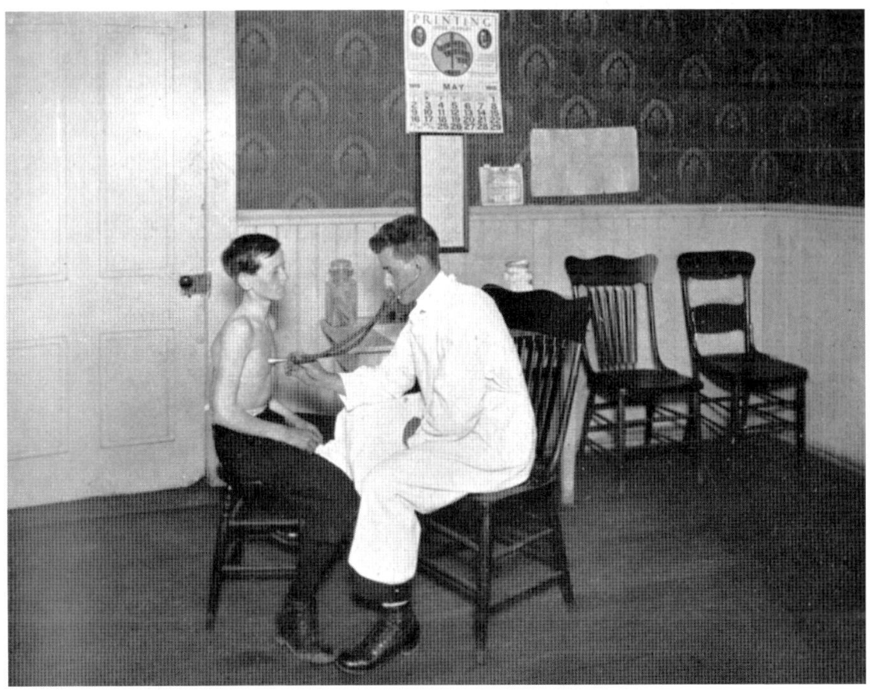
PRINTING
MAY

In early 1908, the Free Tuberculosis Dispensary closed due to lack of funds. It reopened several months later under the management of the Board of Tuberculosis Hospital, allowing the Kentucky Anti-Tuberculosis Association to focus on its educational campaigns.[38] The dispensary provided free tuberculosis examinations to residents of Louisville and Jefferson County. If patients were diagnosed with tuberculosis, they were visited regularly by one of the dispensary's traveling nurses, asked to return to the clinic for checkups, and—once Waverly Hills Sanatorium opened in 1910—put on the waiting list for admission to the sanatorium. The nurses showed patients how to care for themselves and how to protect household members from infection. When tuberculosis deaths occurred, these nurses went back into the homes, "collecting valuable sociological data" and "inspecting the fumigation and rendering assistance and attention whenever needed."[39]

In September 1907, the same year the Kentucky Anti-Tuberculosis Association opened the Free Tuberculosis Dispensary, it also established the first tuberculosis sanatorium in the state. Hazelwood Sanatorium was located just south of what were then the city limits of Louisville and north

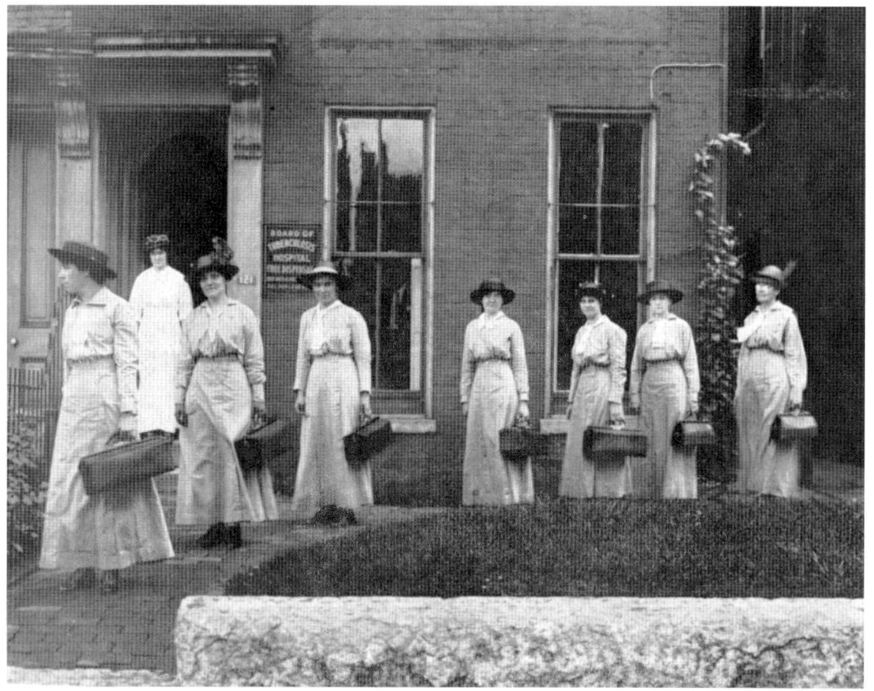

Traveling nurses in front of the Free Tuberculosis Dispensary. Report of the Board of Tuberculosis Hospital, *rare pamphlet 362.16 B662 1916, Filson Historical Society.*

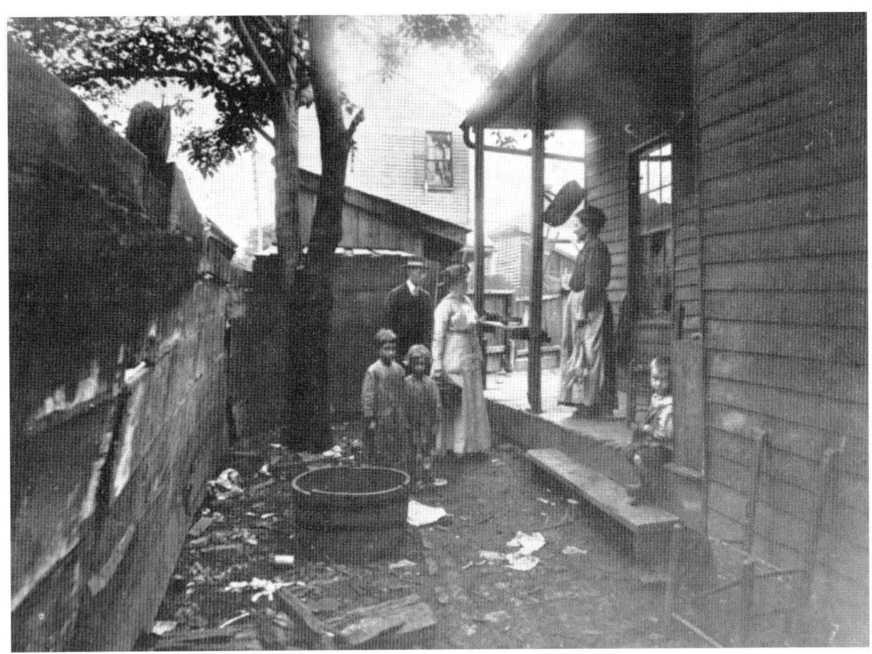

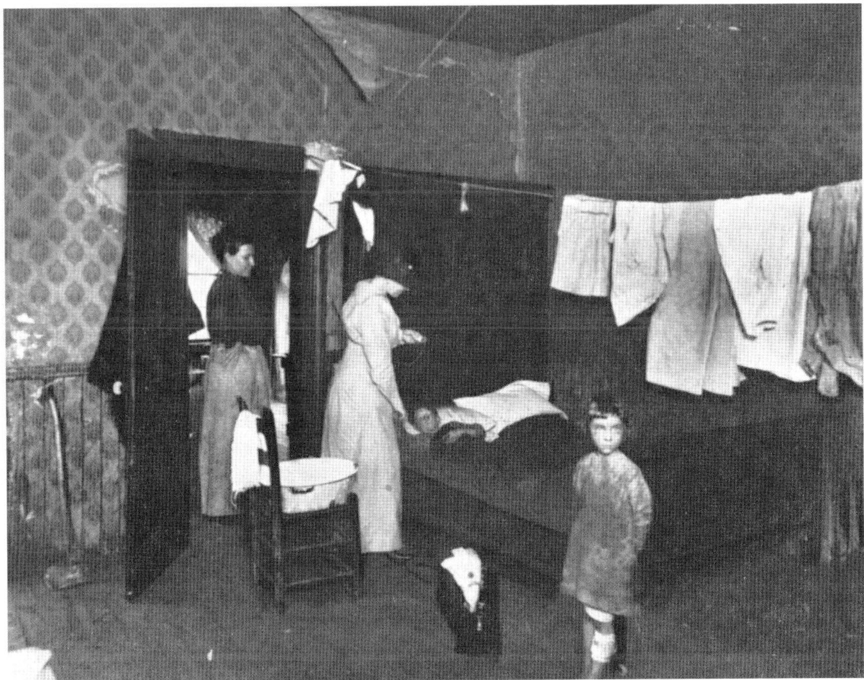

This page: A nurse visiting the home of a tuberculosis patient. Report of the Board of Tuberculosis Hospital, *rare pamphlet 362.16 B662 1916, Filson Historical Society.*

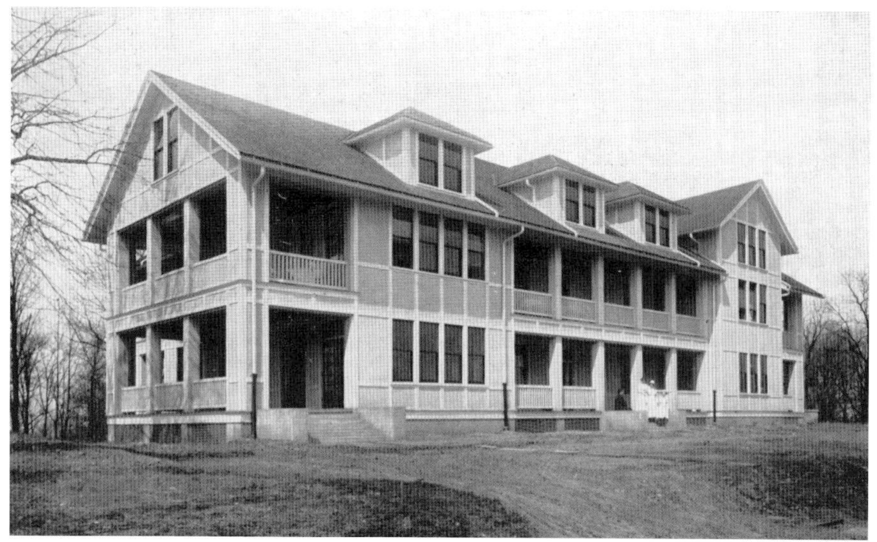

Hazelwood Sanatorium opened in 1907 right outside the city limits of Louisville. *Louisville Anti-Tuberculosis Association,* The Hazelwood Sanatorium, *circa 1917, rare pamphlet 362.16 H429, Filson Historical Society.*

of Jacob Park (later renamed Iroquois Park). It was privately run by the association and provided treatment to white residents of Kentucky for a set fee. According to a pamphlet from the 1910s, the institution helped to meet "the need for a first class sanatorium where any white patient in the State may get treatment and board at actual cost."[40]

Hazelwood was set up along the same model as other tuberculosis sanatoriums of the time. It was located outside the city on the crest of a hill and consisted of a main building, cottages, and tents. The first floor of the main administrative building included a wide porch, a communal living area, a dining room, offices, and living quarters for staff. The second floor had rooms and wards for patients who were mostly limited to their beds. Cottages and tents were reserved for more mobile patients. The grounds had a farm and a dairy; an orchard of apple, peach, cherry and plum trees; and grapevines and raspberry and blackberry bushes. The therapeutic regimen was described as "using as few drugs as possible and depending on the three greatest of nature's remedies, namely rest, fresh air and good food." While some patients were accepted as charity cases, most paid a weekly fee of $12.50 covering "board, medical attention, nursing, ordinary medicines, etc." There was a waiting list for the sanatorium's forty-nine beds.[41]

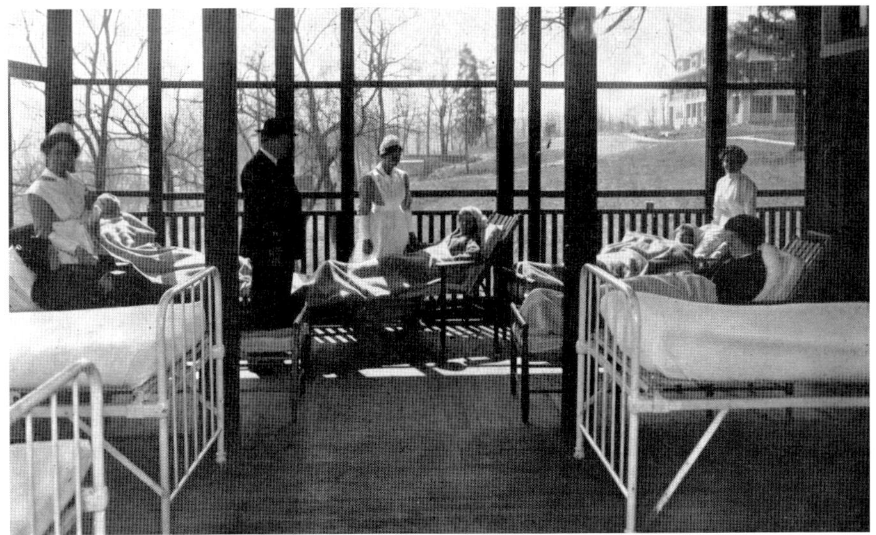

Hazelwood Sanatorium provided treatment to white Kentuckians diagnosed with tuberculosis. *Louisville Anti-Tuberculosis Association,* The Hazelwood Sanatorium, *circa 1917, rare pamphlet 362.16 H429, Filson Historical Society.*

Keeping Hazelwood Sanatorium afloat financially with private contributions proved challenging. A fire burned down the main building in 1912, and the sanatorium closed temporarily in 1914. In 1920, management of the sanatorium passed to the State of Kentucky, and Hazelwood would be run by a state tuberculosis agency until its closure in 1971.[42] Hazelwood's existence as an institution for the treatment of tuberculosis both predated and, as we will see toward the end of this book, ultimately outlived that of Waverly Hills Sanatorium.

Chapter 3

THE FIRST DECADE OF WAVERLY HILLS SANATORIUM

Waverly Hills Sanatorium, while following the same therapeutic principles as Hazelwood Sanatorium, would be a very different sort of institution. From the beginning, Waverly Hills was envisioned as a tax-funded institution providing free board and treatment to white and Black patients from Louisville and Jefferson County, in contrast to Hazelwood's status first as a private sanatorium and then as a state-run sanatorium serving only white Kentuckians. In 1906, W.C. Nones, president of the Kentucky Anti-Tuberculosis Association, said the goal for Louisville's public sanatorium was to construct multiple buildings to separately house "white patients and colored patients" as well as to separate far-advanced cases from early cases of tuberculosis.[43]

Louisville mayor Paul C. Barth, a member of the Kentucky Anti-Tuberculosis Association, initially put forth a much less ambitious plan for the sanatorium. In the fall of 1906, he had plans drawn up for a one-story wood structure with two bathrooms, "one for the colored and the other for white patients," and "four general lounging rooms for the male and female and white and colored patients." He believed the structure could be burned down within five years, when he estimated the sanatorium would accomplish the aim of decreasing tuberculosis rates in the city and county. By the end of the year, however, Mayor Barth had expressed support for the creation of four departments—"white, colored, male and female"—housed in separate and more permanent structures.[44]

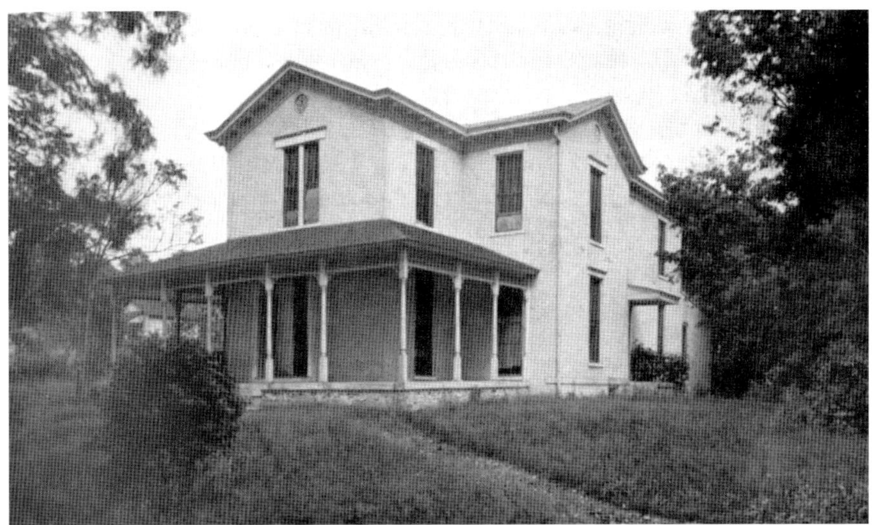

The former home of the Hays family. The house was used at Waverly Hills Sanatorium as a home for nurses. Report of the Board of Tuberculosis Hospital, *rare pamphlet 362.16 B662 1916, Filson Historical Society.*

In January 1908, the Board of Tuberculosis Hospital bought 126 acres on the Waverley Hill property, which had belonged to Major Thomas Hays and his wife, Georgia Hays, since 1883. The name "Waverley" came from Lizzie Lee Harris, a teacher hired by Major Hays for a school he set up for his daughters. Harris named the school after the Waverley novels of Walter Scott, and Major Hays adopted the name for his estate. The property was located in southwest Jefferson County in the Valley Station area, six miles from the Louisville city limits. At its highest point, the Waverley Hill property included views of the surrounding countryside and across the Ohio River.[45]

Immediately after the Board of Tuberculosis Hospital announced the purchase of the Waverley Hill land and the Hayses' home for approximately $20,000, a nearby Valley Station resident filed a lawsuit to stop the sale. Mr. Adams, a farmer, said he feared his family would contract tuberculosis from sanatorium patients. Health leaders and board members defended the purchase. They wanted a location in Jefferson County accessible to passengers of the electric interurban railway lines connecting the center of Louisville to developing suburbs in the county. They wanted access to a railroad for hauling coal and supplies. They wanted enough land for raising cows, chickens, and a garden, as well as a source of fresh water. They looked for "attractive grounds, with trees and picturesque views," since tuberculosis patients spent so much time outside. The Waverley

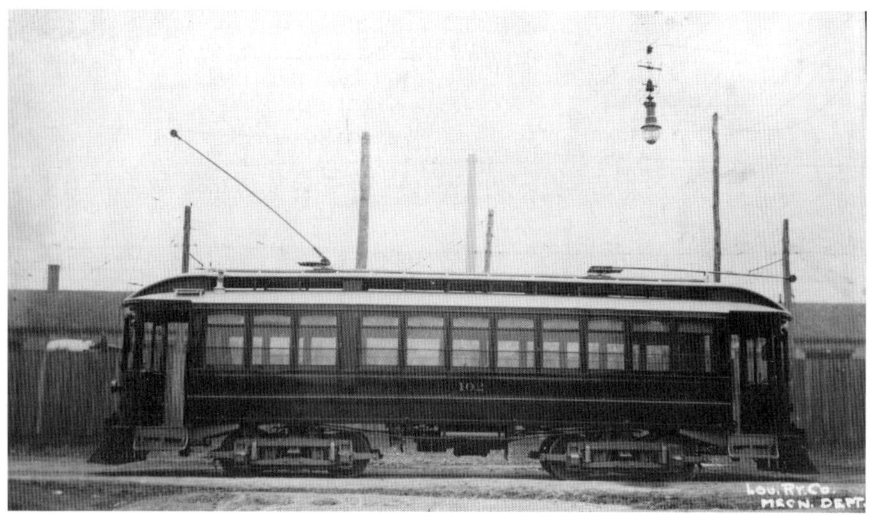

A model similar to this electric interurban car transported patients from Louisville to Waverly Hills Sanatorium. *James B. Calvert Photograph Collection, 988PC71.65, Filson Historical Society.*

Hill property provided all of these qualities at an affordable price. Board members had found "wherever we went that some people were needlessly afraid of the hospital and objected to its location near them," and Waverley Hill was no exception. Unlike the land they had looked at near Anchorage, Jeffersontown, or Crescent Hill, the Waverley Hill property was not located near a settled neighborhood, and it was a mile from Mr. Adams's house. The Orell interurban line had been completed in April 1907, enabling plans to be made for a dedicated electric railway car to transport tuberculosis patients to a stop near the sanatorium.[46]

Despite continued opposition from Valley Station residents, the board moved forward and hired local architect J.J. Gaffney to design the $150,000 sanatorium. Plans for multiple facilities for different groups of patients required more funding than what was available. Instead, the original sanatorium consisted of a two-story stucco administration building flanked on each side by an open-air pavilion, each with twenty beds and enclosed bathing facilities and dressing rooms. The administration building served as the "center of operations" for the sanatorium. The first floor included the offices of the medical director and the superintendent of nurses, a laboratory, chart and drug rooms, the medical and nursing staff dining room, and a classroom for nurses. The second floor housed living quarters for the nurses. The back part of the building was occupied by the patients'

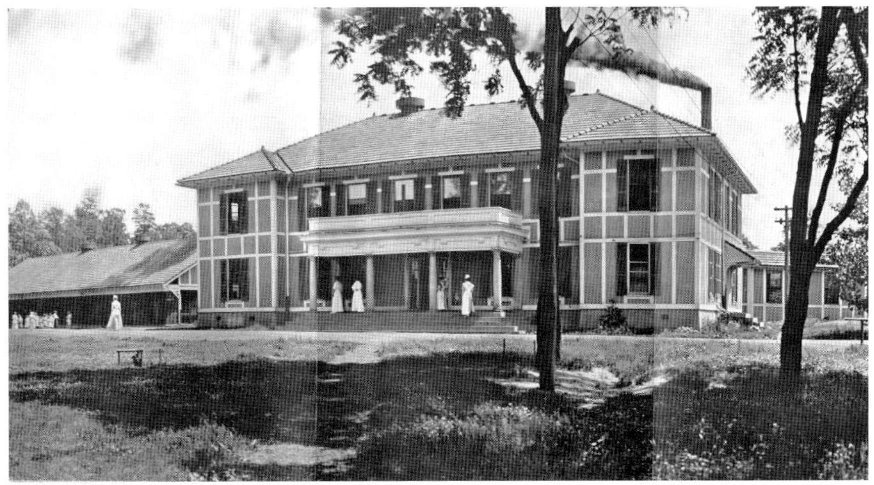

The Waverly Hills Sanatorium administration building and two pavilions opened in 1910. Report of the Board of Tuberculosis Hospital, *rare pamphlet 362.16 B662 1916, Filson Historical Society.*

and the employees' dining rooms, the kitchen, the storeroom, and an ice refrigeration room. In the basement were the laundry and living quarters for other employees.[47]

Waverly Hills Sanatorium opened to patients on July 26, 1910, with the formal dedication on October 12. At this early point, only white patients with early cases of tuberculosis were admitted. The south pavilion housed male patients and the north pavilion female patients.[48] Dr. A.M. Forster served as the first superintendent and medical director of Waverly Hills but resigned in November 1910. Taking his place was Dr. Dunning Wilson, who had previously served as superintendent of Hazelwood Sanatorium. He would remain at the helm for six eventful years, during which Waverly Hills would expand its facilities and capacity to over 250 beds.[49]

THE HOSPITAL FOR ADVANCED CASES

In 1910, the only facility for advanced cases of tuberculosis in Jefferson County was a thirty-five-bed tuberculosis annex to the City Hospital, Louisville's public general hospital dating back to the early nineteenth century. In early 1911, all of City Hospital's patients were being moved into temporary quarters and out of the old hospital building about to be torn down, making way for a new $1 million hospital with duplicate, racially segregated facilities. Officials announced in March that when the construction of the new City Hospital was completed, it would no longer admit any tuberculosis patients.[50]

Taken aback by the City Hospital announcement, the Board of Tuberculosis Hospital pressed the city for funds for a hospital for advanced cases of tuberculosis at Waverly Hills. Mayor William O. Head called for a $25,000 appropriation. After the city funds were approved, patients were moved in August 1911 from the City Hospital tuberculosis annex to temporary tents at Waverly Hills. The patients remained in the tents while the new hospital at Waverly Hills was constructed during the next year and a half. The tents were described as "substantial" and were erected on raised wooden floors, with temporary buildings to the rear outfitted as bathrooms. Dr. Wilson later recalled those months as "trying times of caring for these patients…during the vicissitudes of weather both fair and foul, both hot and cold." He said the tents increased the capacity at Waverly Hills to ninety beds, including "the far advanced and white and black of both sexes."[51]

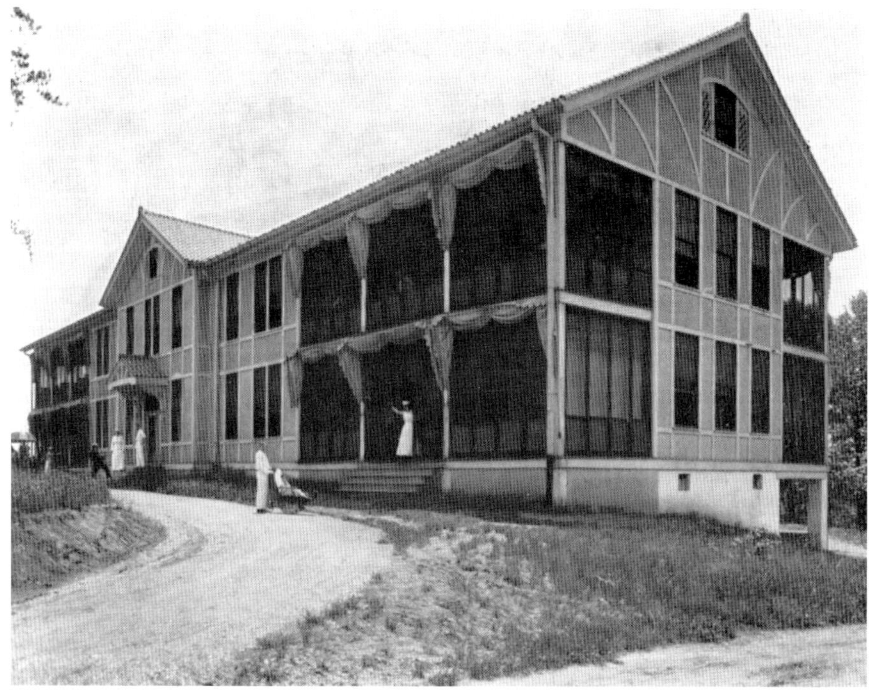

The hospital for advanced cases at Waverly Hills opened in January 1913. Report of the Board of Tuberculosis Hospital, *rare pamphlet 362.16 B662 1916, Filson Historical Society.*

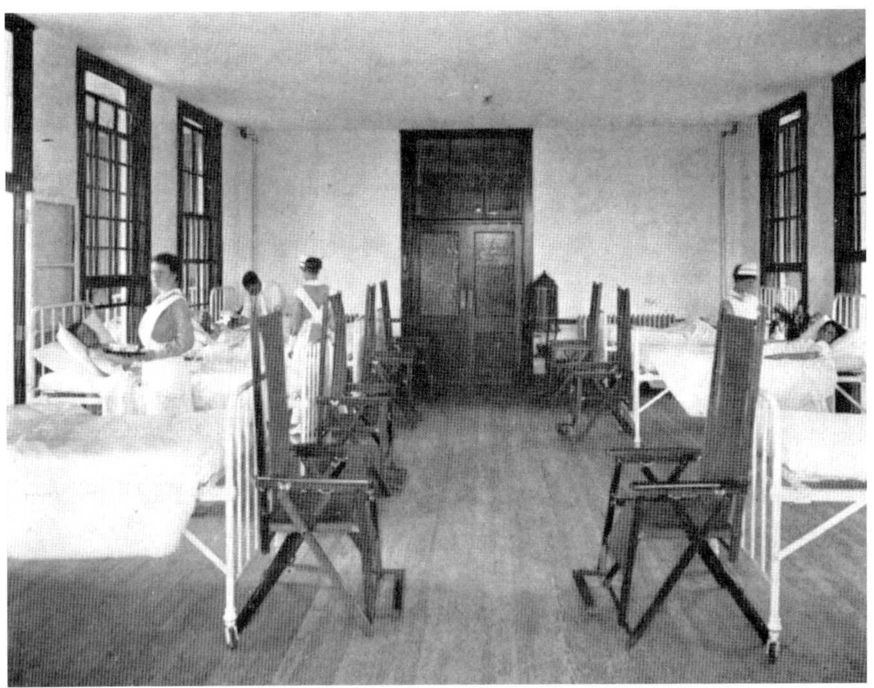

White female patients in a ward of the hospital for advanced cases. Report of the Board of Tuberculosis Hospital, *rare pamphlet 362.16 B662 1916, Filson Historical Society.*

J.J. Gaffney, who designed the original Waverly Hills administration building and pavilions, was hired again to make plans for the hospital for advanced cases. The two-story, half-timbering wood frame building with a hipped roof opened in January 1913 with fifty beds.[52] The patients housed in tents walked or were carried over a quarter mile to the new hospital, located downhill from the original buildings on another high point on the grounds. The *Courier-Journal* described the hospital as nestled in its natural surroundings, with spacious quarters segregated by gender and race:

> *The bright tile roof of the new hospital gleams around the first curve of the long winding roadway that climbs the sanatorium hill, and is the brightest spot on the beautiful landscape that spreads out about the Waverly Hill property. The building has two large open wards on each floor, four wards in all, providing a very satisfactory separation of the sexes among both white and colored patients, all of whom can gaze out from the wards over wonderful panoramas of the river country to the north and the broken hills toward the south.*[53]

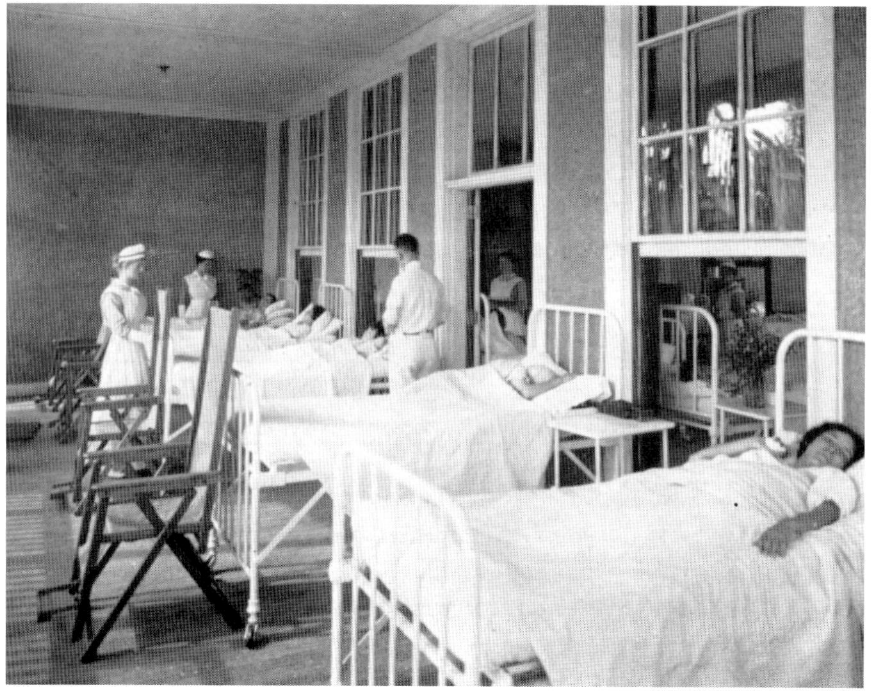

White female patients on a porch of the hospital for advanced cases. Report of the Board of Tuberculosis Hospital, *rare pamphlet 362.16 B662 1916, Filson Historical Society.*

By 1914, total capacity at Waverly Hills had increased to 170 beds located in the original pavilions (which continued to house white patients with early cases of tuberculosis), the hospital for advanced cases (which held white and Black patients), and additional cottages and temporary accommodations. According to the Board of Tuberculosis Hospital, just over 1,000 patients were admitted to the sanatorium from July 1910 through September 1914. Of this total, 251 were Black and 757 were white, and 635 were categorized as far advanced cases. In these first four years, a total of 322 patients died at Waverly Hills, and patients with far advanced tuberculosis accounted for nearly all the deaths.[54] These numbers serve as a stark reminder of how deadly tuberculosis was in the 1910s for patients in the advanced throes of the disease—a point this book will return to in the last chapter.

A SCHOOL AND PAVILION FOR "PALE LITTLE FOLK"

In addition to building the hospital for advanced cases, Waverly Hills officials were focused on providing new accommodations for children in the early 1910s. According to Dr. Dunning Wilson, no hospital in Louisville accepted children with tuberculosis, who deserved better care than what they received in the "squalid surroundings" of the city. Before the children's pavilion opened in 1916, children were housed at Waverly Hills in the adult quarters. Dr. Wilson said that adult patients saw the children as "nuisances" ("and they are," he added). He wanted to move children into their own housing to open up beds for adult patients and to help relieve a long waiting list.[55]

A makeshift open-air school served sixteen white children at Waverly Hills at the end of 1911. A *Courier-Journal* article touted the open-air school as a haven for "pale little folk of the city who coughed," referring to the pallid countenance of patients with tuberculosis. The article chronicled the treatment of a boy named Albert, painting an idealized picture of outdoor life and schooling for children at the sanatorium. Albert had been taken by a tuberculosis nurse from his home and deposited "kicking and screaming" on the interurban car to Waverly Hills. During his first three months at the sanatorium, Albert was transformed from a frail, sick child to a happy, rosy-cheeked one, sleeping on an open porch, taking three hearty meals a day, and visited often by his mother.[56]

The school was conducted on the end of the porch of the women's pavilion. The children were arranged in a semicircle from the lowest grade level to the most advanced, all facing the teacher, Dena Woodward. In cold weather, there was no heating apparatus but only blankets, layers of clothing, and hot water bottles to keep the children warm. The students were sent to take a nap from one to three o'clock every afternoon, followed by a snack of "a big bowl of milk with crackers." They sat for another hour of school and then took part in gentle afternoon recreation. Boys made bird and squirrel boxes for the school garden, and girls were taught how to make their beds and mend their clothes. Rather than expressing sorrow for these patients, the *Courier-Journal* article asked readers to think about the children who never got to enjoy such fresh food and air: "Pity the child who never knew to cut his name on some old tree, who never romped through sun and shade, nor rested on the rugged roots of some great oak or elm and felt the cooling breath that moved beneath its branches—the child of hot streets and shut-in homes, where stale air and strong disease kept company!"[57]

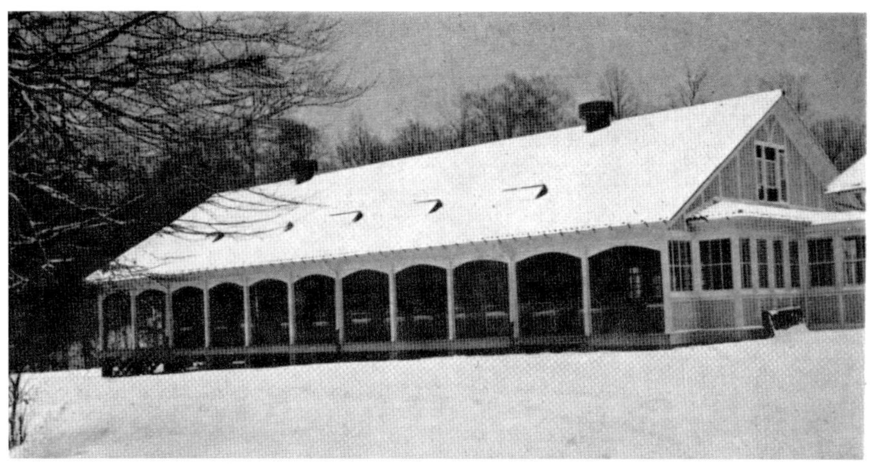

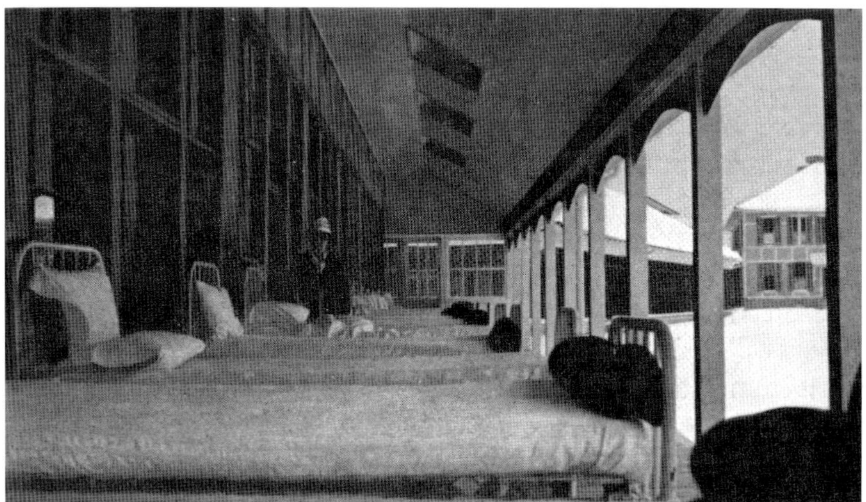

This page: The children's pavilion at Waverly Hills Sanatorium was equipped and ready for patients in 1916. Report of the Board of Tuberculosis Hospital, *rare pamphlet 362.16 B662 1916, Filson Historical Society.*

With the help of journalistic boosterism, carnival fundraisers, and increases in the city's tax levy for the sanatorium, the money was secured for the construction of a children's pavilion in 1915. By the spring of 1916, additional funds had been raised to furnish and staff the pavilion, and it was ready for patients. At this point, the Jefferson County Board of Education took over formal management of the school at Waverly Hills, and administration was shared with the Louisville Board of Education beginning in 1919.[58]

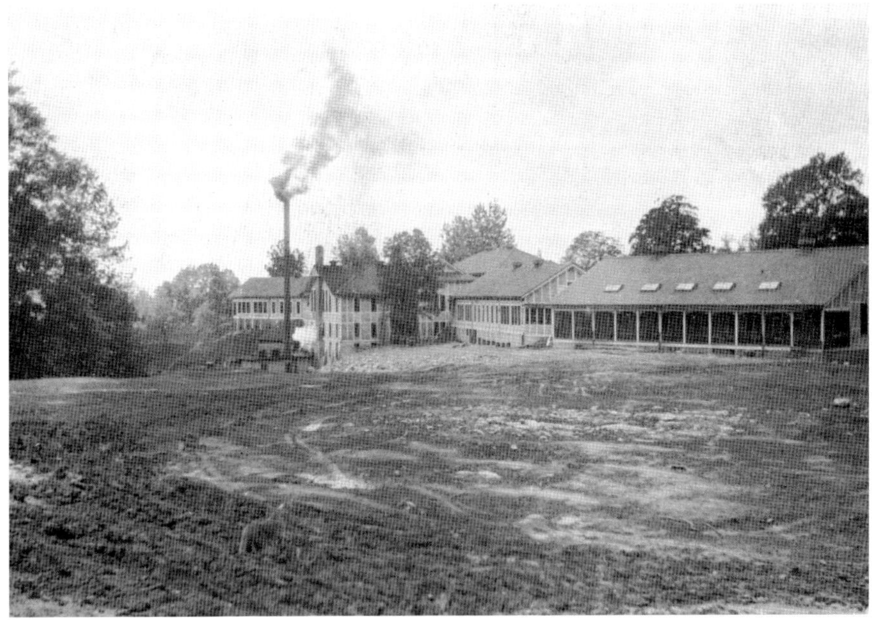

The back side of the original administration building and pavilions, including the children's pavilion on the right, circa 1920s. *Edward Arthur Waverly Hills Photograph Collection, 019PC9.17, Filson Historical Society.*

Both the new children's pavilion and the Waverly Hills School served only white children. In the 1910s and first half of the 1920s, Black children admitted to Waverly Hills were evidently housed along with Black adults in the hospital for advanced cases. In addition to not making space for Black children in the children's pavilion, the Board of Tuberculosis Hospital and city and county officials also failed to provide formal schooling for Black children during these years. Kentucky's 1904 Day Law prohibited mixing "white and colored persons" in any public or private schools, from the elementary grades to graduate programs. For Black children at Waverly Hills, this meant there was no city- or county-run school at all.[59]

While there is little information about the number or experiences of Black children treated at Waverly Hills, the pavilion for white children remained at capacity. In 1919, a reported 60 percent of the children admitted to Waverly Hills Sanatorium were "suspects"—children who did not have symptoms of tuberculosis but were suspected of harboring a latent or an "incipient" (early) form of the disease due to their exposure to an adult with tuberculosis in their household. Officials could not compel adult patients to seek treatment at Waverly Hills, but an order of the court gave them

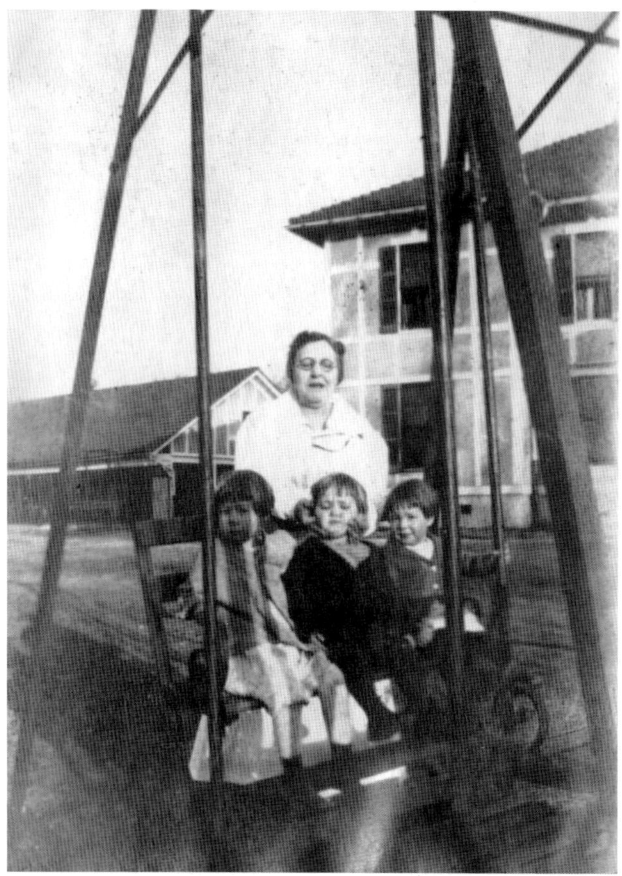

Left: A nurse with children on a swing at Waverly Hills, circa early 1920s. *Edward Arthur Waverly Hills Photograph Collection, 019PC9.26, Filson Historical Society.*

Below: Children in chairs on the grounds of Waverly Hills, circa early 1920s. *Edward Arthur Waverly Hills Photograph Collection, 019PC9.26, Filson Historical Society.*

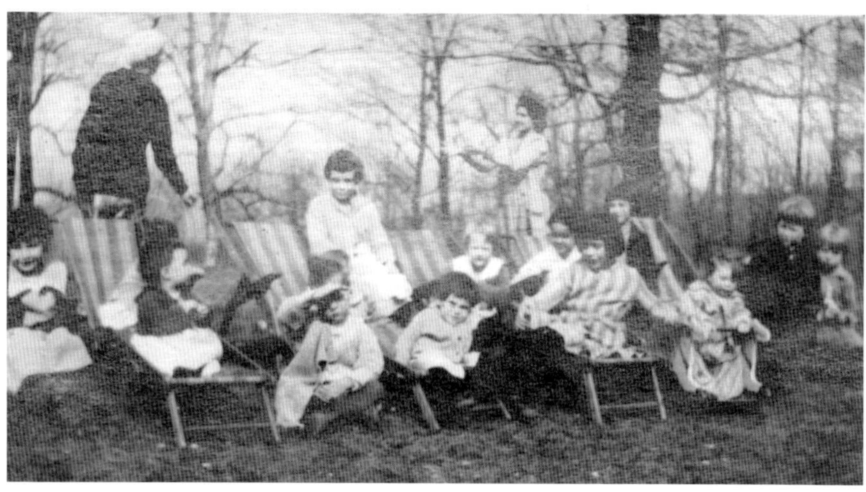

the authority to remove children from homes where they had been exposed to tuberculosis. The children could be placed at Waverly Hills if officials deemed family members incapable of providing a "proper home" for them or if their parents were hospitalized at the institution. The *Courier-Journal* claimed this was a positive arrangement, helping the children to overcome a possible bacterial infection: "The chances are good for the prevention of the disease if they remain at the sanatorium long enough. Such a merry, happy bunch of little folks as they are!"[60]

Fighting for Health at Waverly Hills

The number of patients at Waverly Hills Sanatorium during the first decade was constantly in flux with the addition of temporary and permanent accommodations. A 1916 national directory of sanatoriums listed Waverly Hills as having a capacity of 255, with "102 advanced cases in Hospital; 103 up cases in Sanatorium; children's pavilion, 50."[61] The hospital for advanced cases had been built to hold just 50 beds but, according to this listing, was housing twice as many patients. The "sanatorium" referred to the original pavilions meant to hold 40 beds total but likely also included additional cottages and tents helping to boost the capacity for "up cases" (patients who were not limited to their beds) to 103 patients. It is not clear where all of these patients were living at Waverly Hills, but it is certain the pavilions and wards were crowded.

In 1911, before the opening of the hospital for advanced cases, new arrivals to Waverly Hills were immediately put to bed and remained there until they went six consecutive days without a fever. Once new patients were fever-free for six days, they became an "up patient." Patients at the sanatorium took part in the following routine:

> *At 6:30 o'clock the first whistle blows, and the patients tumble out of their beds, wash, dress and get ready for breakfast, which is served at 7 o'clock. The bed patients' meals are brought to them on a tray which sits up on the bed. After breakfast the nurses take temperatures, respiration, and pulse. At 10 o'clock a glass of rich certified milk is drunk, and at 12:30 dinner is served. From 1 until 3 o'clock bed patients and up patients alike must sleep, or, if they can't sleep, remain quiet on their bed, so others can sleep. At 3 o'clock milk again, after temperatures have been taken. Supper is at 5:30 o'clock and temperatures again. When a patient has a temperature of 99.6*

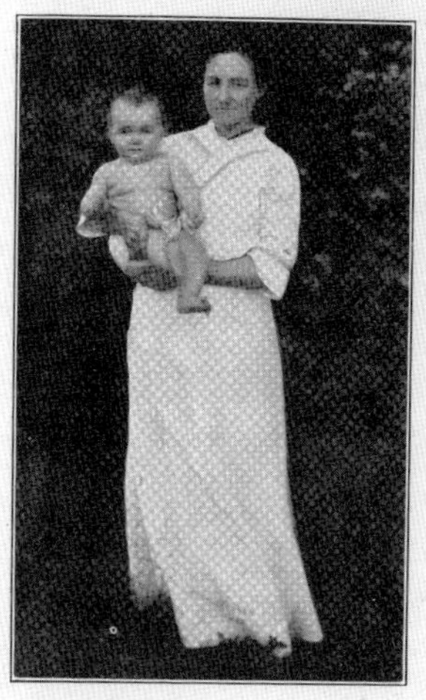

First
Baby Born
at
Waverly Hill.

The mother who is seen here holding her infant had thirty-three hemorrhages before admission. When admitted she was hemorrhaging and was in a precarious condition. Her child was born prematurely about six weeks later. Under the care of the institution she is regaining her health.

Is This Work Worth While?

Left: The first baby born at Waverly Hills. Report of the Board of Tuberculosis Hospital, *rare pamphlet 362.16 B662 1916, Filson Historical Society.*

Below: Men on the porch of the pavilion at Waverly Hills, circa early 1920s. *Edward Arthur Waverly Hills Photograph Collection, 019PC9.26, Filson Historical Society.*

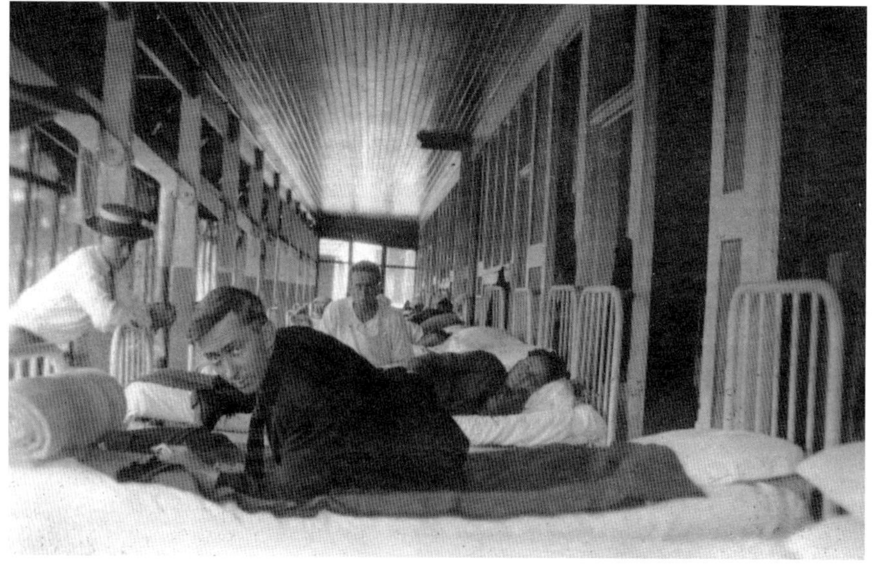

> *he is put to bed until three consecutive normal days have been registered. At 9:15 o'clock the lights all over the building are "flashed" and are turned off fifteen minutes later, when the patients must all be in bed. After supper those who desire can remain in the dining room until 9 o'clock and talk or play games that do not require exertion.*[62]

The highly regulated routine of Waverly Hills Sanatorium was difficult for patients to endure. The sanatorium prohibited alcohol and tobacco, with "no exceptions made," but many patients and employees through the years illicitly sold and consumed liquor. In the early years of Waverly Hills, patients were allowed to leave the sanatorium to visit home for the day once every six weeks if they were physically well enough to do so, but many patients simply left and stayed home. Louisville health officials called for a law to keep "advanced cases from leaving the institution, thereby doing themselves injury, and at the same time leaving a trail of infection wherever they go." However, no legislation compelling hospitalization of adult patients was passed until the mid-1950s.[63]

Beds were a significant expense for a medical institution in which the main form of treatment was rest. In the first several years of Waverly Hills Sanatorium, furniture and bedding made up almost two-thirds of

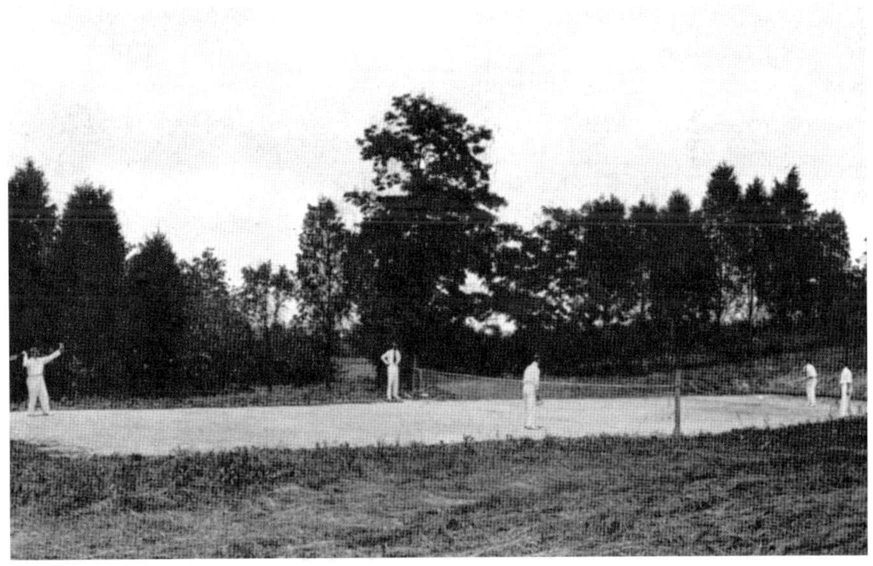

The tennis court for medical staff at Waverly Hills. Report of the Board of Tuberculosis Hospital, *rare pamphlet 362.16 B662 1916, Filson Historical Society.*

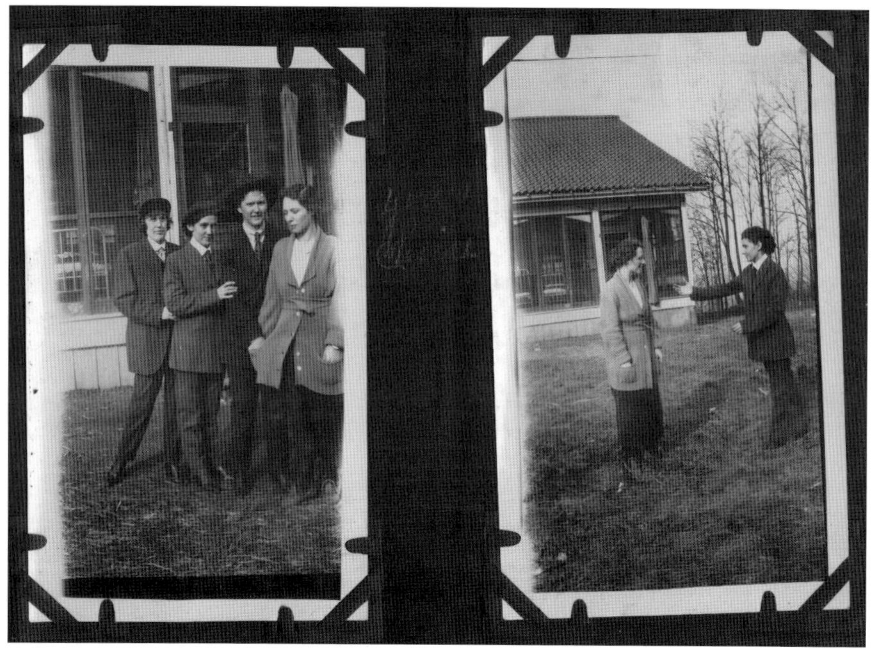

Young women dressed up as men and posing with another young woman in front of a pavilion at Waverly Hills. *Edward Arthur Waverly Hills Photograph Collection, 019PC9.26, Filson Historical Society.*

equipment costs. From 1910 to 1914, as the sanatorium was increasing the number of beds, $8,400 was spent on furniture and $9,600 on linen and bedding. During those same years, only $890 was spent on medical and surgical equipment, about the same amount of money spent on horses and mules, harnesses, and farm implements. The farm provided fresh produce to patients, who were given vegetables at every meal, as well as a steady diet of milk, eggs, and meat. Officials called for the establishment of a dairy and hennery at Waverly Hills so the sanatorium would not have to continue to buy large quantities of milk and eggs.[64]

In addition to the established trilogy of rest, fresh air, and nutritious food, Waverly Hills offered newer technologies and procedures. Although X-rays were still in the early decades of development, they were becoming an important part of diagnosing tuberculosis and monitoring the effects of the disease in the lungs. In 1921, the *Courier-Journal* reported that new X-ray equipment had recently been installed at the hospital for advanced cases. Heliotherapy (exposure to the sun) and artificial heliotherapy (exposure to a sun lamp) were seen as modern treatments, especially for patients suffering

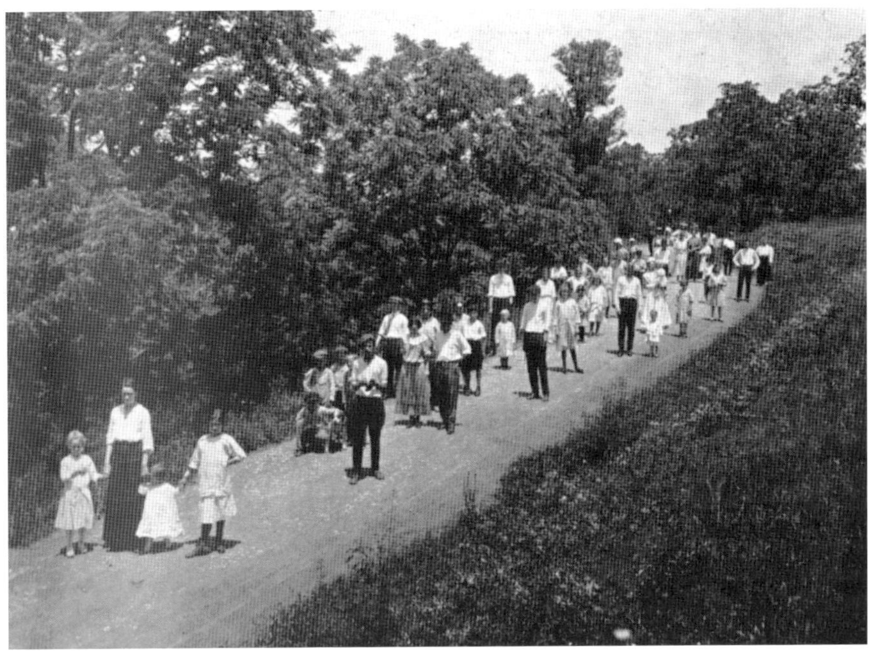

Exercise hour at Waverly Hills Sanatorium. Report of the Board of Tuberculosis Hospital, *rare pamphlet 362.16 B662 1916, Filson Historical Society.*

from tuberculosis of the bone and joints. Artificial pneumothorax, involving the injection of air by needle into the pleural cavity to force the patient's diseased lung to collapse temporarily and give it time to heal, was gaining popularity among physicians treating tuberculosis.[65]

Nursing care remained a critically important part of the treatment of tuberculosis throughout the history of Waverly Hills Sanatorium. To help provide a supply of nurses, the Board of Tuberculosis Hospital established a training school for white female students in 1912. The school was affiliated with the Louisville City Hospital Training School for Nurses. According to Dr. Dunning Wilson, the training program would prepare nursing students not just for positions at Waverly Hills Sanatorium but also for "missionary and sociological work outside the hospital, in preventing the spread of the disease." As the number of beds at Waverly Hills and patients on the waiting list increased, so did the need for more nurses at the sanatorium and at the Free Tuberculosis Dispensary. The dispensary's corps of traveling nurses was seen as "the only means of defense against infection from those who do not come to the institution."[66]

TONICS AND SEDATIVES

SCENES AT WAVERLY HILL

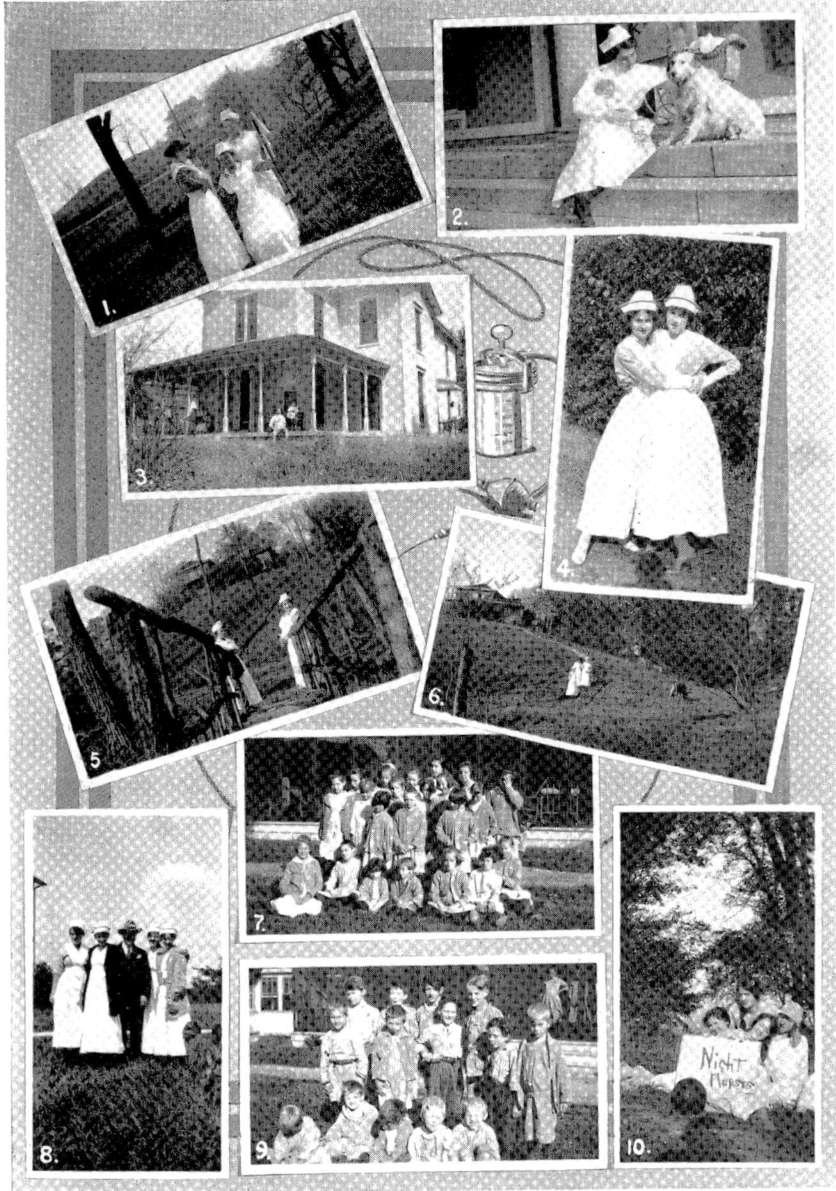

Nursing students at Waverly Hills Sanatorium. Tonics and Sedatives, *Louisville City Hospital Training School for Nurses, 1919, Kornhauser Health Sciences Library, University of Louisville.*

The outbreak of the First World War in 1914, with the United States entering the war in 1917, posed new challenges to the provision of care at Waverly Hills Sanatorium. Dr. Dunning Wilson resigned in the summer of 1916 to enlist in the Kentucky National Guard. After a short interim during which the twenty-seven-year-old Dr. J.B. Floyd served as medical director and superintendent, Dr. Oscar O. Miller took the position in 1918.[67]

The devastating influenza epidemic of 1918 struck Louisville in the fall. Just outside the city limits was Camp Zachary Taylor, one of the largest military cantonments constructed in the United States during the war. The enormous size of the camp, with over forty thousand soldiers, officers, and staff, meant infectious diseases could spread quickly. On September 24, Louisville newspapers reported that more than one hundred soldiers at the camp had been diagnosed with influenza. On September 27, a quarantine prohibited soldiers from traveling into the center of the city, but the disease had already begun to spread. As cases of influenza increased rapidly in Louisville in early October, tuberculosis and public health nursing associations joined together to provide traveling nurses and trained volunteers to help care for influenza patients in their homes. A statewide closure of churches, schools, and recreational places was put into place until cases began to drop in the last few weeks of October. A second increase in cases following Thanksgiving led to more closures.[68]

For nursing students at City Hospital who had just finished their training at Waverly Hills in mid-September, the influenza epidemic meant "no hours, no half days off duty—Just work, work, work. Nurses off duty—sick—they have got the 'flu.'" The strain may have contributed to the closing of the nurses' training program at Waverly Hills in November 1918. After this point, Waverly Hills relied on other nursing schools, such as City Hospital's, for nursing students and graduates.[69]

Waverly Hills Sanatorium emerged from the end of the war and the influenza epidemic to face other problems. A growing waiting list included many veterans who had contracted tuberculosis during the war. The hospital for advanced cases was already considered a fire hazard that the Board of Tuberculosis Hospital hoped to replace soon. Asked in 1921 about what was still needed at the sanatorium, the editor of the *Waverly Hill Chronicle* focused on more lighthearted wants and called for more flowers and a swimming pool.[70]

Chapter 4

A NEW SANATORIUM AND A NEW DIVISION

Health leaders and advocates in the 1920s publicized the ongoing fight against tuberculosis, highlighting falling death rates and a growing acceptance of sanatorium treatment among middle-class as well as working-class patients. They cited statistics from 1918–19 showing over two-thirds of patients diagnosed with tuberculosis followed their physicians' advice to go to Waverly Hills Sanatorium for treatment and claimed "the class of patients seeking admission has raised." Yet officials reported that Kentucky still had the second-highest death rate from tuberculosis among states in the country. Instead of California, now only Colorado—another "tuberculosis mecca"—had a higher death rate from the disease.[71]

In early January 1922, Waverly Hills officials proposed a $750,000 bond issue to fund the construction of a new $1 million sanatorium building, with the bond issue to be put before the voters on election day in November. The current Waverly Hills facilities reportedly had a mammoth-size waiting list of 2,600 individuals. The hospital for advanced cases was an overcrowded "fire trap." Board of Tuberculosis Hospital president A.H. Bowman described the wretched condition of the hospital's wards: "Patients are crowded together in an insanitary and inhuman manner because of the lack of room. The negro ward is so congested that only the sexes are separated and the children and adults are thrown together, as also is the case with far advanced and incipient patients." Grand juries charged with inspecting the facilities at Waverly Hills reported only one bathroom for every 25 patients, porches being used as permanent bed space, and inadequate surgical facilities.[72]

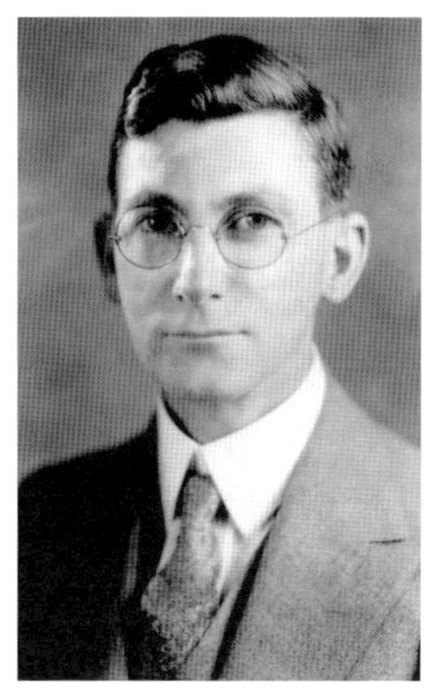

Dr. Oscar Miller served as medical director and superintendent of Waverly Hills Sanatorium throughout the 1920s. *ULPA 1994.182792, Archives and Special Collections, University of Louisville.*

Leading up to election day in November 1922, many different groups mobilized to raise support for the proposed bond issue. Louisville Women's City Club members sold tickets to an "air circus" at Bowman Field (an airfield opened in 1922 by board president Bowman) and emphasized the need to provide treatment to veterans who had contracted tuberculosis during the war. Organizers also drew attention to the "impoverished" condition of Waverly Hills Sanatorium and the continued lack of cows or chickens, even though fresh milk and eggs were "the principal diet of tubercular patients" (Waverly Hills, it seems, never got its cows or chickens). The army provided pilots for the June 17 air show, which ended tragically when aviators Lieutenant Robert O'Hanley and Sergeant Arthur Opperman crashed during a low-flying maneuver and were killed. The two men were memorialized as giving their lives both "in the service of their country and in the cause of fighting tuberculosis."[73]

As the November 7 election approached, other advocates for Waverly Hills implored voters to approve the bond issue for the sake of children and adults in need. The *Courier-Journal* printed an image of white children in beds crowded on the children's pavilion porch. A caption stated that more than fifty of the two hundred patients at Waverly Hills were children, with many more waiting for treatment.[74] The Welfare League took out a large advertisement in the newspaper to make a "mighty appeal for the poor, unfortunate, needy, suffering ones of our city":

> *Suppose your doctor said:—"You have tuberculosis but proper care and attention will save you—and you haven't the money to buy this care and attention, you could get it without cost at Waverly Hills but unfortunately there is no room there"—let us prevent this dreadful situation by voting "yes" on Tuesday for the WAVERLY HILL BOND ISSUE—Afflicted humanity calls you to vote, "Yes."*[75]

On November 7, the hospital bond issue was carried by the voters "almost unanimously." The $750,000 bond issue plus a $250,000 appropriation by

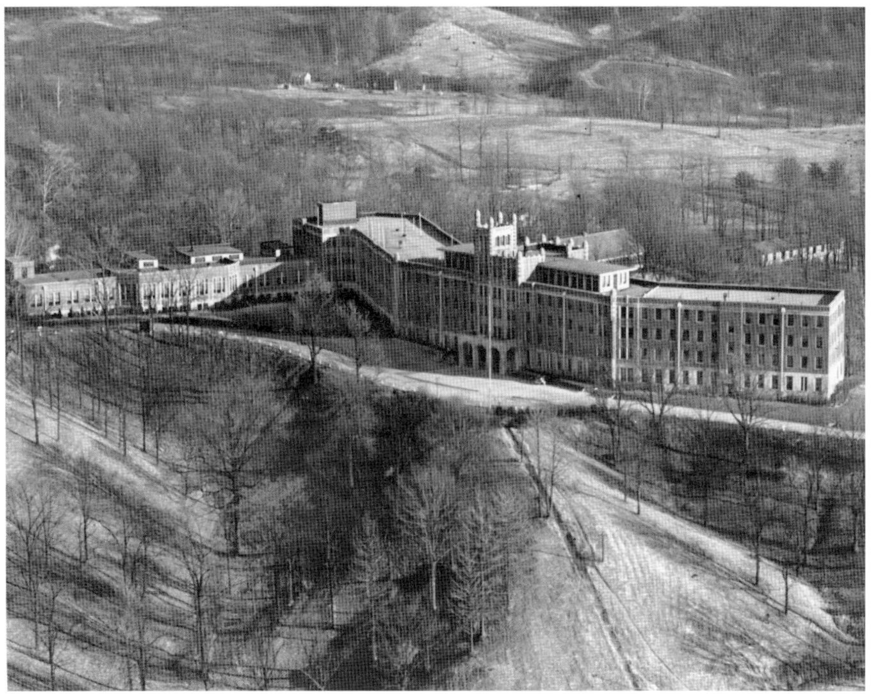

Aerial view of the main sanatorium that opened in 1926. *Courtesy of* Louisville Courier-Journal.

the county provided the funds needed to build and furnish "a modern and completely equipped million dollar hospital" at Waverly Hills. Arthur Loomis was hired to design the new sanatorium, and D.X. Murphy's architectural firm assisted and oversaw construction. Final plans were for a fire-resistant, four-story brick and stone building in the Tudor Gothic Revival style and the shape of an irregular semicircle. The building plans included a partial fifth floor, a square tower, and a three-bay arched entrance.[76]

The groundbreaking took place on May 12, 1924, next to the original administration building and the pavilions. The administration building and women's and children's pavilions would be connected to the new sanatorium building, with the administration building converted into an auditorium and staff accommodations. The men's pavilion was moved just south of where the new sanatorium was built and refurbished as quarters for male employees.[77]

The new sanatorium building was constructed to hold 400 beds, two to each room. At its opening in 1926, only 286 beds were available to patients, with the rest of the rooms used as living quarters for nurses. The partial fifth floor housed the heliotherapy ward for patients suffering from tuberculosis of the bone. Other facilities located in the building were a laboratory, an X-ray room, a surgical suite, kitchens with refrigerated storerooms, a bakery, laundries, and an occupational therapy department. Also included were amenities of all sorts "for the comfort and amusement of the patients." There was a recreation room with a stage for plays and a screen for movies, a chapel, a library, a barbershop, and a beauty parlor. The south-facing side of the wings on the second through the fourth floors had communal sun porches running the length of the building. Patient rooms on the south side had doorways through which beds could be wheeled onto the porch. The rooms on the north side of the building were reserved for patients too physically frail and sick to be wheeled outside. Every bed in the new building was equipped with an audio radio attachment.[78]

Completed in September 1926, the new sanatorium had its formal dedication ceremony on October 20. Dr. Lawrason Brown, a prominent tuberculosis expert from the Adirondack Cottage Sanatorium in New York

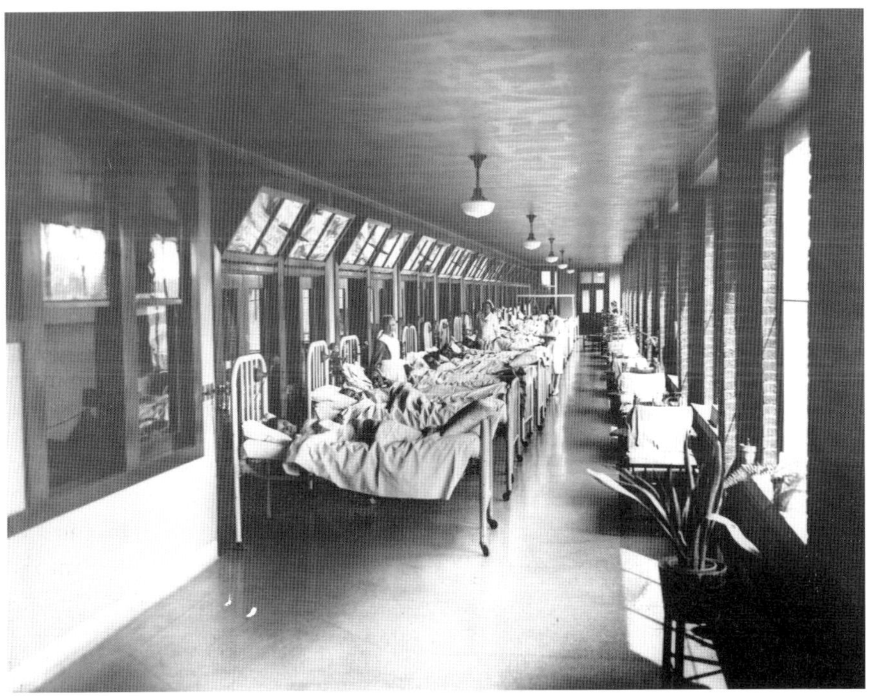

One of the long sun porches on the south side of the main sanatorium. *Courtesy of* Louisville Courier-Journal.

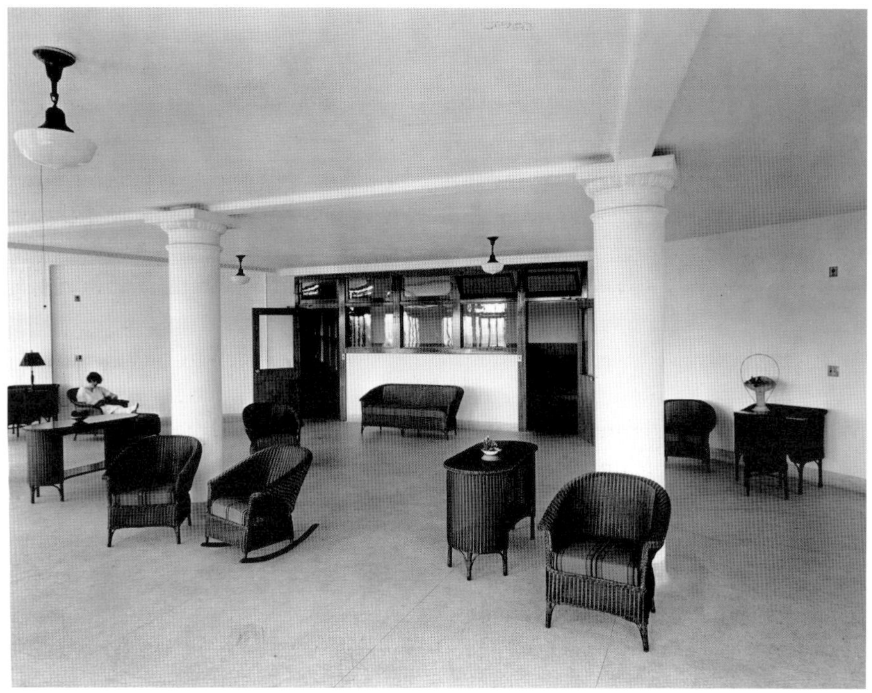

One of the solariums in the main sanatorium. *Courtesy of* Louisville Courier-Journal.

who served as consultant for the new building's design, gave the main address. He told the audience, "Tuberculosis may no longer be called the captain of the men of death, but it stands shoulder to shoulder with the other captains, and the fight into which it has plunged medicine has led to a broad struggle to improve the public health."[79]

A RENOVATED HOSPITAL FOR BLACK PATIENTS

Unlike the $1 million City Hospital that opened in 1914 and provided racially segregated facilities, the new $1 million Waverly Hills building that opened in 1926 provided no beds or even segregated wings for Black patients. The accommodations and amenities of what was called the "main sanatorium" at Waverly Hills were for white patients only.

A history written in the 1950s, attributed to Louisville Tuberculosis Association rehabilitation director Catherine Richardson, pointed to the opening of the new sanatorium in 1926 as an event leading to other significant developments: "Those who had planned this imposing new building, looked across the landscape and saw new visions. A home for nurses, a new hospital for colored patients, residences for staff physicians, and steady improvements in techniques and equipment." This statement was partly true. A new dormitory-style building was constructed to house white nurses in 1929, and three new brick homes were built as private residences for physicians and their families. But the "new hospital for colored patients" was actually the old hospital for advanced cases, with some unspecified renovations.[80]

To raise support for the 1922 bond issue for the new sanatorium building, white officials had courted Black voters, as they had also done with a $1 million bond issue for the University of Louisville that led to the establishment of the Louisville Municipal College for Black students in 1931.[81] Dr. Archibald C. McIntyre, a Black physician in Louisville who went on to serve in leadership positions in state and national medical organizations, later reminded *Courier-Journal* readers of Black voters' support for the Waverly Hills bond issue: "The colored citizens of Louisville and Jefferson County were promised and assured that a colored department would be established providing for the employment of a colored resident physician, nurses and helpers."[82] In 1924, a survey of Louisville hospitals confirmed what was already well known: Louisville's hospitals, most of which excluded Black patients, nurses, and physicians, provided far fewer beds per capita for Black patients and "wholly inadequate clinical opportunities" for Black medical professionals. In 1925, after the bond issue had passed and the new sanatorium was being built, the Interracial Commission of Kentucky added its voice in the call for "a resident Negro physician and nurses for Negro patients" at the "new Tuberculosis Sanatorium at Waverly Hills."[83]

Upon the opening of the new sanatorium in 1926, white patients housed in the pavilions took up residence in the new building, and then white patients from the hospital for advanced cases were transferred. Histories from the 1950s identify "eleven Negro patients" who were temporarily moved while the hospital for advanced cases underwent renovations to turn it into a facility exclusively for Black patients. In April 1927, the multiple buildings of Waverly Hills housed a total of 361 patients, 39 of whom were "men and women at the Colored Hospital."[84] Earlier in the 1910s and 1920s, *sanatorium* had denoted the part of Waverly Hills treating patients with early or moderate cases of tuberculosis. *Hospital* was the term for the facility treating white and Black patients with advanced cases who needed more intensive care, although the Black wards of the hospital

Louisville has twelve hospitals, one for tuberculosis and eleven general hospitals of which eight admit white patients only, one, the City Hospital, serving both white and colored, and two hospitals for colored only:

Hospital Facilities of Louisville

	Number of Beds	
Public Institutions—		
Louisville City Hospital (White and Colored)	418	
Waverly Hill Sanatorium (White and Colored)	210	
		623
Voluntary Institutions—		
Baptist Hospital	146	
Children's Free Hospital	72	
Deaconess Hospital	65	
Fraternal Hospital (Colored)	30	
Jewish Hospital	74	
Norton Memorial Infirmary	110	
Red Cross Sanitarium (Colored)	38	
St. Anthony's Hospital	170	
St. Joseph's Infirmary	100	
Sts. Mary & Elizabeth Hospital	145	950
Total		1,573

The number of beds and patients served at each hospital in Louisville and Jefferson County. *Haven Emerson and Anna C. Phillips,* Hospitals and Health Agencies of Louisville 1924: A Survey, *65.*

mixed patients with both early and advanced cases. After 1926, the use of the name *sanatorium* for the new building for white patients and the name *hospital* for the facility for Black patients seemed to serve the purpose of further distinguishing between the two racial divisions of Waverly Hills rather than characterizing the severity of cases treated in the different buildings.

A Black graduate nurse and eventually a Black physician were hired to oversee the care of patients at the Black hospital. Esther M. Barrens began working as nurse supervisor in the hospital in August 1926. The white physician Dr. Alvin B. Mullen, who had joined the Waverly Hills medical staff in July, took charge of white patients on the third floor of the main sanatorium and supervised Barrens in her work at the Black hospital. The Waverly Hills administration had a hard time hiring and retaining Black nurses at the hospital, a problem largely due to the paucity of training programs for Black nursing students in Kentucky and the low pay for practical nurses who were trained on the job. Barrens was sometimes the only nurse on duty in the Black hospital in the years to come. In 1927, Dr. Henry W. Bond of Louisville was the first physician hired at the hospital. Dr. Orville Ballard, the son of a pharmacist in Lexington, took over Dr. Bond's position at the hospital in 1928 after Bond resigned.[85]

In 1928, local Black physicians commended the creation of positions for Black staff at Waverly Hills, but they also noted the substandard condition of the Black hospital. Dr. Archibald McIntyre described the growth of the Black division during its first eighteen months as "phenomenal" but also as overcrowded and underequipped. "Upon a visit to the institution," he wrote, "one is impressed with the cheerfulness which apparently pervades the situation, and a congenial well-fed, though poorly and unsanitarily quartered group of inmates who greet you at every turn." The number of Black patients had increased from eleven to over seventy in a hospital meant

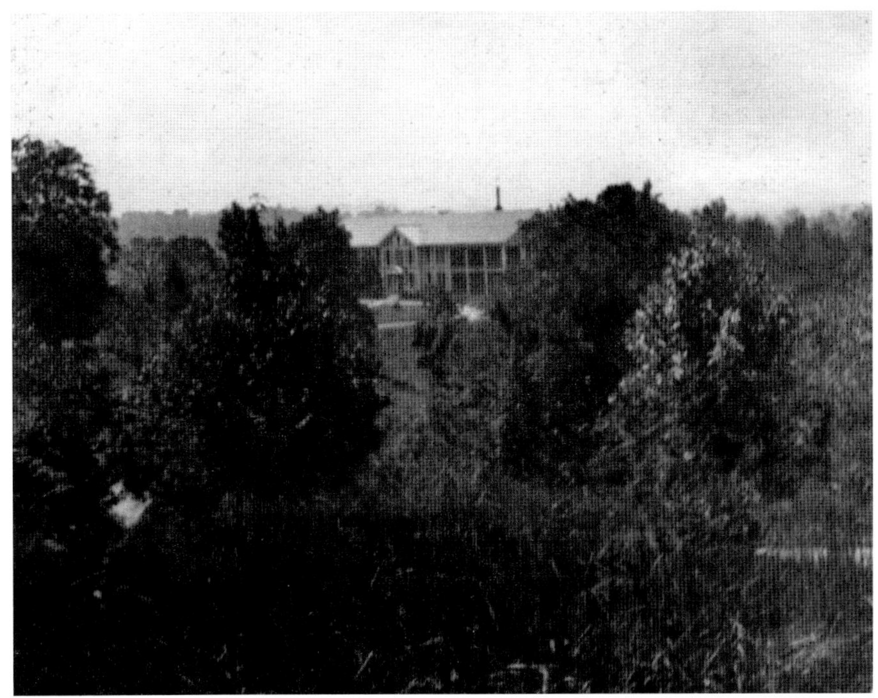

View (from the location of the main sanatorium) of the hospital for advanced cases that became the Black hospital in 1926. *Edward Arthur Waverly Hills Photograph Collection, 019PC9.26, Filson Historical Society.*

to house fifty, with a long waiting list for beds. Despite these problems, Dr. McIntyre said the employment of Black medical staff at Waverly Hills and at a public clinic in Louisville had boosted the willingness of Black patients to seek sanatorium treatment. "The whole attitude and atmosphere," Dr. McIntyre wrote, "has been changed in regard to Waverly Hills Sanatorium on the part of the colored people." More early cases were being admitted, and more patients were remaining at the institution for the full duration of their treatment. Before the hiring of Black employees, "dissatisfaction on the part of patients" limited their stay to three or four weeks at most. Now many were willing to stay for "several months or more."[86]

Dr. McIntyre and other Black leaders in Louisville formed a "Citizens Committee," which lobbied the Board of Tuberculosis Hospital to address the need for Black representation on the board and for improvements to the Black division at Waverly Hills. They presented the following petition to the board at its meeting on July 17, 1928:

> *The Citizens Committee recommends the appointment of a Negro representative to serve on the governing board of Waverly Hill Sanitorium, selected upon the recommendation of the Citizens Committee. We recommend maintenance and beginning salary for a resident physician the sum of $150 per month. Improvement of the living quarters of the physician and nurses separate from the main institution if possible; better recreational facilities and educational advantages for the children; some occupational therapy that will aid convalescent and tend to lessen stay in in the sanitarium.*

The petition was signed by Dr. McIntyre, Reverend G.F. Watson, J.M. Ragland, Reverend Reynolds, I. Willis Cole (publisher of the *Louisville Leader*), Dr. J.H. Walls, W.H. Stewart, and Dr. Bond.[87]

A Black representative was not appointed to the Board of Tuberculosis Hospital, and board members and administrators took decades to incrementally expand accommodations and services for Black patients and employees. Without the same level of resources or staffing provided to white patients in the new sanatorium, Black Louisvillians took matters into their own hands. In 1927, the City Federation of Colored Women's Clubs raised money to update bathrooms at the Black hospital. In the late 1920s, nurse supervisor Esther Barrens initiated elementary-level classes for children and taught needlework to adult female patients, attempting to make up for the lack of a city- or county-run school for Black children at Waverly Hills and the lack of a properly staffed occupational therapy program for Black adult patients.[88]

LETTERS FROM THE SANATORIUM

Firsthand accounts of what it was like to be a patient living at Waverly Hills, especially at the Black hospital, are scarce. Merrill Montgomery and Stella Hatfield are two white patients whose letters from the main sanatorium from 1928 to 1930 have survived. Montgomery wrote letters to his friend from Hazelwood Sanatorium and one from Waverly Hills Sanatorium seven months before he died there. Stella Hatfield, who was in her mid-twenties and about five years younger than Montgomery, wrote a series of letters during two years of her time at Waverly Hills, ending five months before her death at City Hospital.

Born in Seymour, Indiana, Merrill Montgomery graduated from Hanover College in 1914. He traveled to Hollywood, California, to work in the silent movie industry and returned to his home state by 1920. In letters to his childhood friend Lynn Faulkoner, Montgomery wrote of seeking treatment at tuberculosis hospitals in Cincinnati, Ohio, and at Saranac Lake, New York, in the early 1920s and then at Hazelwood Sanatorium and Waverly Hills Sanatorium in 1927–28. At the state-run Hazelwood Sanatorium in Louisville, he wrote of nurses regularly taking his temperature, heart rate, and weight. When his fever "popped up to 102.2" and his heart rate increased in early August 1927, he had to limit himself to the bed but used a wheelchair "as a means of Locomotion." By his next letter, he had successfully gained 4 pounds, putting him at 110¼ pounds, "so there is plenty of room for more gain."[89]

Toward the end of 1927, Montgomery noted the loss of "those precious four pounds," which he blamed on the stress of his relations with women at Hazelwood. As he reported to Faulkoner, "A girl went down to the cottage where the nearly well patients are and spread a lot of apple sauce about me and there was a stampede of women up here. It was too much

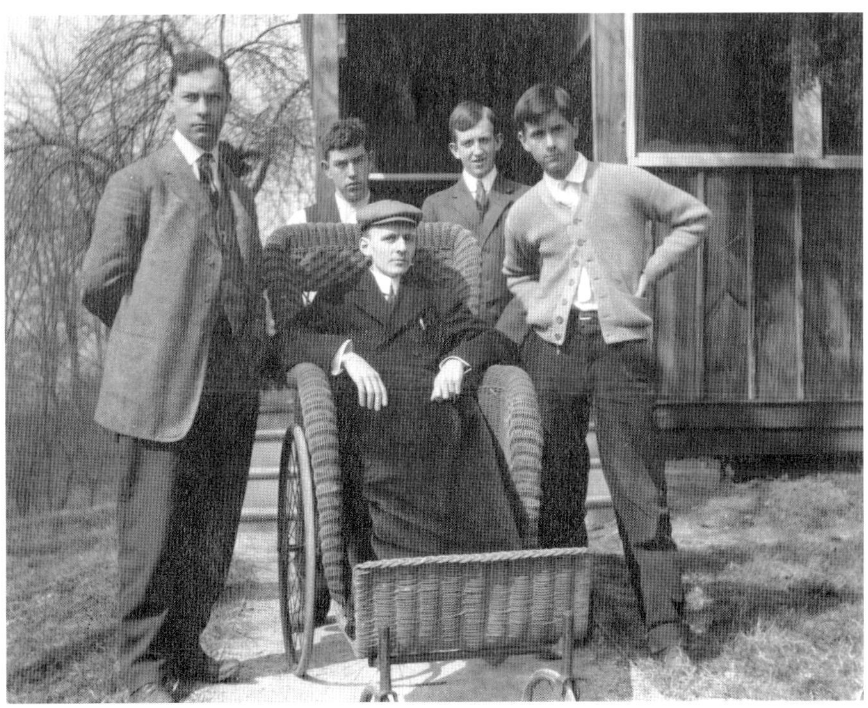

Many tuberculosis patients used wheelchairs for mobility. In 1927, Merrill Montgomery wrote of using a wheelchair during his time at Hazelwood Sanatorium. *Edward Arthur Waverly Hills Photograph Collection, 019PC9.16, Filson Historical Society.*

for me I guess." He declared the experience "amusing" but asked, "Why in the devil did they pick on a bird so helpless as me is clear beyond my understanding." After the female patient he liked "better than all the rest" was reprimanded by a physician for being upstairs where she was not supposed to be, Montgomery was finding his days "much quieter" and was hoping for improvement in his health.[90]

While Montgomery was at Hazelwood, he was plotting ways to gain admission to Waverly Hills, which he said was a "much finer institution."[91] Writing Faulkoner from Hazelwood late in the summer of 1927, he detailed all the attributes of the new sanatorium at Waverly Hills:

> *It is brand new, a million Dollar Bldg. all the latest equipment, better Doctors and everything and there they have a private room for every two patients where you can be pulled in when the weather's too cold, you're not well or want to entertain company, tho you're on a long porch with maybe 50 others most of the time. There is a radio at the head of every bed. Dr. Lawrence* [sic] *Brown the best at Saranac was out here and spent some time getting them started right and is medical adviser. Oscar Miller the best T.B. Doctor in Louisville or Kentucky is at the head of it.*

Montgomery noted that Waverly Hills was free to Jefferson County residents and charged twenty-five dollars a week to people from outside the county, but the sanatorium currently had no beds for nonresident paying patients.[92]

It took Montgomery over a year to gain admission to Waverly Hills, a feat he accomplished in late August or early September 1928. In a long letter written from Waverly Hills on September 20, he told Faulkoner his condition had worsened at Hazelwood, where he lost twenty-three pounds over the spring and summer. It had taken him six months to set up an official residence for himself at 1271 Everett Avenue in Louisville, and his father and a friend had to "pull the wires with the Mayor of Louisville" to get him into Waverly Hills. The mayor called Dr. Oscar Miller on Montgomery's behalf, and within twenty-four hours, a nurse told Montgomery that he could go right over to Waverly Hills. Montgomery described Mayor William B. Harrison as "one real fine fellow, about 29 years old, and handsome enough to be a movie star," who came out to see him at the sanatorium soon after he was admitted. Montgomery asked Faulkoner to keep secret that he was from Indiana and that he had received help from the mayor, as "they are very strict about entrance" at Waverly Hills. He used a derogatory, racist term to refer to the Black hospital at Waverly Hills, as he claimed the racial privileges of free treatment at the main sanatorium for white patients.[93]

Montgomery was one of many patients from outside the county and the state trying to finagle their way into Waverly Hills Sanatorium in the late 1920s. In March 1928, about six months before Montgomery was admitted, the Board of Tuberculosis Hospital prohibited for a period of one year the admission of all nonresidents of Louisville and Jefferson County, including those who moved into the city and county limits to live with relatives. In response to the number of people who set up residence for themselves to gain admission to Waverly Hills, the board in October 1929 declared a preference in admissions for residents who had lived in the city or county their whole lives. The president of the board said, "We have at Waverly Hills what seems to be a perpetual waiting list."[94]

Montgomery's September 20, 1928 letter detailed the many treatments and services he received during his first several weeks at Waverly Hills, showing why so many patients from beyond Jefferson County tried to gain admission to the sanatorium. There was "a whole flock of Doctors" at the main sanatorium, with one to two physicians assigned to each floor. During his first several days, the physicians took blood and sputum samples for tests and X-rayed his chest, stomach, and intestines. They examined his sputum every day for the first ten days, but the tests all came back negative for tuberculosis. It is unclear whether Montgomery ever received a firm diagnosis of tuberculosis during his years of treatment at different sanatoriums.[95]

Waverly Hills physician Dr. Benjamin Brock told Montgomery that the medical staff would discuss his case and would likely want to perform a phrenectomy—what Montgomery called "the nerve operation." No other letter exists to confirm whether he underwent the procedure. A phrenectomy involved crushing the phrenic nerve connected to the diaphragm. By disabling the part of the diaphragm on the side of the diseased lung, physicians aimed to temporarily collapse the lung to prevent bacteria from multiplying and to give the lung a chance to heal. Over a period of months, the nerve repaired itself and resumed control of the diaphragm. A phrenectomy was one of several forms of lung collapse therapy. Other procedures were artificial pneumothorax, which Waverly Hills physicians had been performing since the 1910s, involving the use of a needle to inject air into the chest cavity and requiring refills of air over a period of months. Thoracoplasty involved the removal of several ribs to permanently collapse the diseased lung. These procedures often resulted in less sputum production and thus were seen as ways of controlling the spread of tuberculosis both inside and outside of

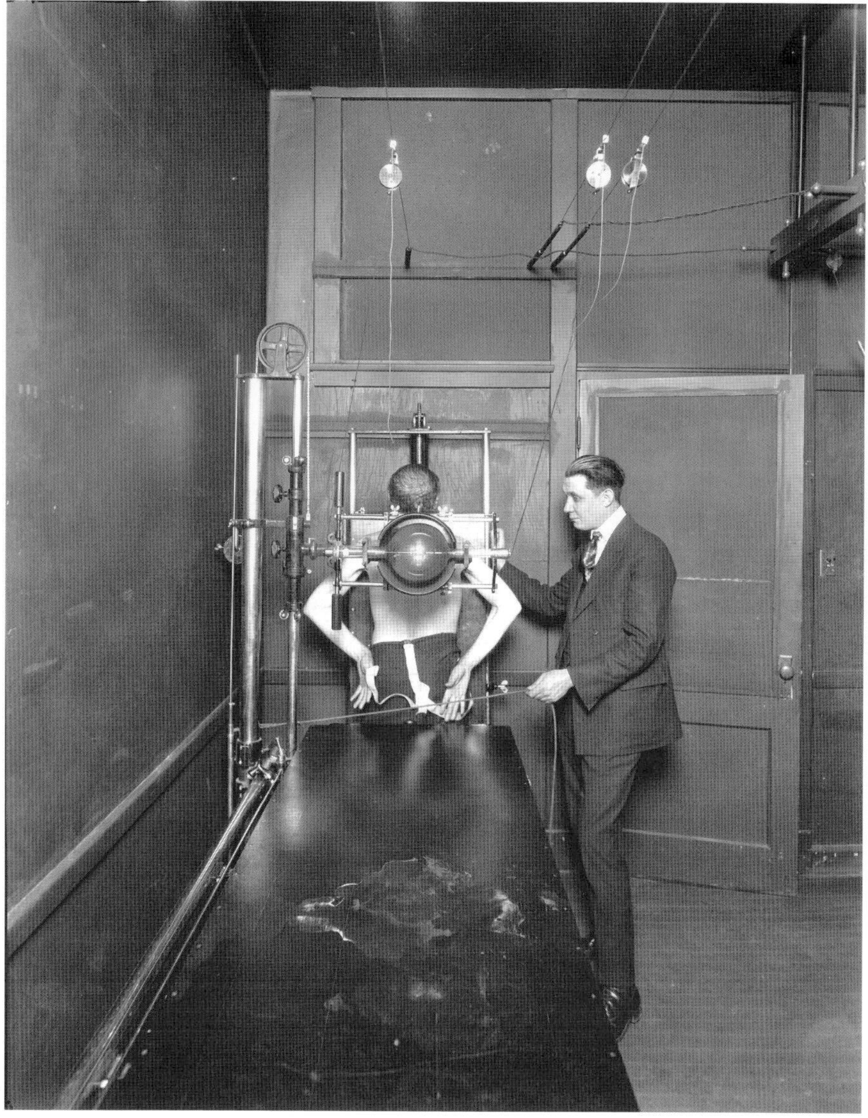

A physician using an X-ray to examine a patient at Waverly Hills, circa 1910s-1920s. *Caufield and Shook Collection, 40463, Archives and Special Collections, University of Louisville.*

patients' bodies. Like other surgical procedures, however, they carried risks of pain and complications. Scarring in the lung and reduced lung capacity could cause other respiratory problems.[96]

Montgomery wrote of benefiting from the fresh air and food at Waverly Hills, enabling him to gain almost five pounds in his first few weeks even

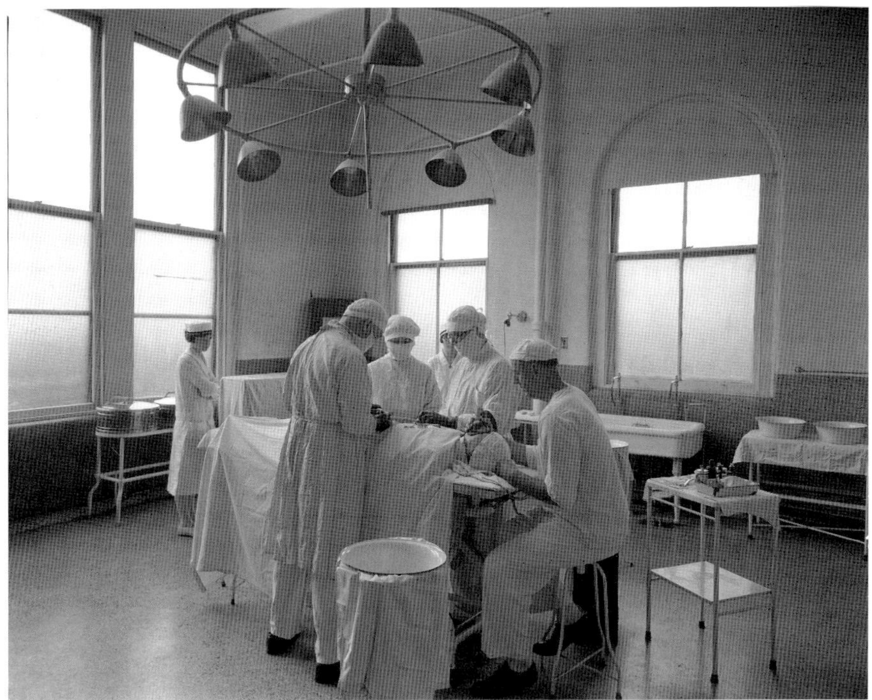

An operating room at Waverly Hills Sanatorium, 1928. *Caufield and Shook Collection, 87031, Archives and Special Collections, University of Louisville.*

though he said he still looked like a skeleton. He had "a ravenous appetite," he told Faulkoner, and the food was "much better here" than at Hazelwood. He ate large meals and drank twelve glasses of milk a day. His bed on the sun porch had "a beautiful view of numerous hills, that looks like Adirondack country." In addition to eating and resting, he spent some time socializing with fellow patients on his floor: "all the fellows seem congenial and we have a pretty good time," and many men played cards, checkers, and craps. Opportunities to mingle with the female patients, who lived on the second and fourth floors of the sanatorium building, were limited mainly to the main dining room or the theater, "and you have to be in pretty good shape to go to either." He asked Faulkoner to come see him at the sanatorium during one of three visiting days—Tuesdays and Thursdays from 3:00 to 5:00 p.m. and Sundays from 2:30 to 5:00 p.m.[97]

Montgomery told Faulkoner that Waverly Hills gave him "some hopes" for recovery, but he died there the following year on May 5, 1929. His age on his death certificate is identified as "about 30 unknown" and his residence as 1271 Everett Avenue in Louisville. The names of his parents and birthplace were listed as "unknown," but Waverly Hills staff evidently made contact with his family, as Montgomery's place of burial was recorded as his hometown of Seymour, Indiana. The cause of death was identified not as pulmonary tuberculosis but as chronic interstitial pneumonia with a duration of fifteen years and a contributing factor of malnutrition over the past four months.[98]

Stella Hatfield's time at the main sanatorium at Waverly Hills from 1929 to 1930 partially overlapped with the months Merrill Montgomery was there. For Montgomery, writing letters was a way to reach out to his friend and to process the progression of his disease and treatment. Stella Hatfield's letters were written not to a friend or family member but to the assistant of Robert Worth Bingham, a prominent lawyer, politician, and owner of the *Courier-Journal* and *Louisville Times* newspapers. Bingham was a founding member of the Kentucky Anti-Tuberculosis Association. He had taken on Hatfield as a charity case and had directed his assistant Emily Overman to send Hatfield checks every month and to respond to her requests for things she wanted or needed at Waverly Hills. Hatfield never wrote to Overman of her own family, and her death certificate, like Merrill Montgomery's, listed her father and mother as unknown.

Stella Hatfield suffered from tuberculosis of the bone. Her case affected the joints in her hips and the bones of her legs, shortening one of them, causing her pain, and restricting her ability to walk. At Waverly Hills, her bed was located in a ward on the partial fifth floor of the main sanatorium. Her ward housed white female patients with tuberculosis of the bone, and they received heliotherapy on the roof on sunny days. Hatfield often noted her "three hours sun treatment each day the sun shines." In an early February 1929 letter to Overman, Hatfield reported that her hip was doing better and that she was able to walk "all over the ward" by holding on to furniture.[99]

Hatfield asked Overman to send her a varied list of items. She often requested clothing and shoes, including black patent leather slippers, belts, bloomers, and flannel pajamas and a robe for sleeping outside during the winter months.[100] In March 1929, she asked for a ukulele and an instruction book, a request tinged with sadness. She told Overman how other girls at the sanatorium had ukuleles. She wanted one to "keep me from getting blue" when she was "up here all alone" on the fifth floor on visiting days, while patients gathered with family members in other parts of the sanatorium building. Overman sent Hatfield a ukulele soon afterward. By mid-April, Hatfield said she had learned twenty-five chords.[101]

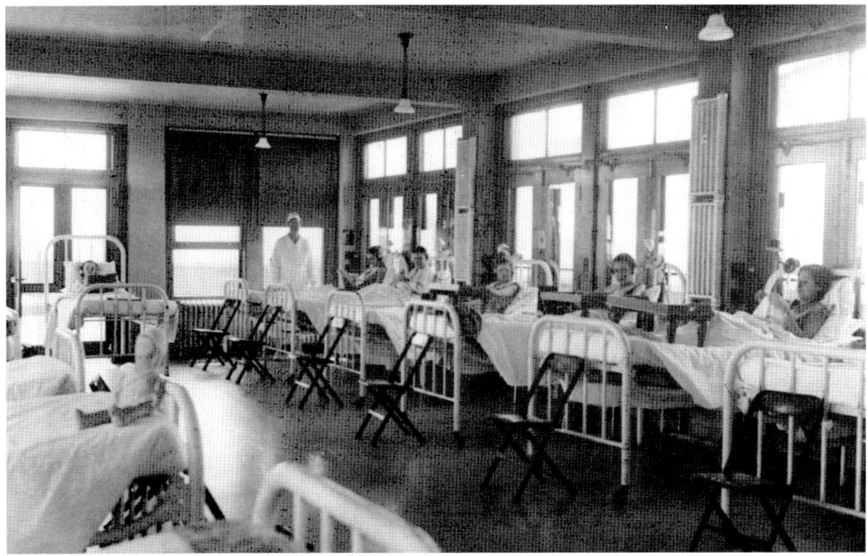

A women's ward at Waverly Hills Sanatorium, 1935. Stella Hatfield wrote of her ward on the main sanatorium's partial fifth floor, which housed patients with tuberculosis of the bone. *Courtesy of* Louisville Courier-Journal.

Hatfield wrote frequently about her time doing occupational therapy and taking art classes, and she asked Overman for specific fabrics, sewing materials, and art supplies. The occupational therapy program at Waverly Hills dated back to the early 1920s, with physicians "prescribing" what sorts of activities patients could take part in and for how long each day. Patients made rugs, baskets, wicker tables, toys, doll houses, sweaters, and carved bookends, keeping some of the finished products for themselves. Other goods were sold and the profits split between the patient and the sanatorium, with potential buyers assured that all articles had been thoroughly sterilized. The main sanatorium included an entire shop area devoted to occupational therapy, which Hatfield referred to as the "O.T. shop."[102]

Over the course of Hatfield's letters to Overman, she provided updates on both her physical condition and emotional state. In the summer of 1930, she seemed to sink to one of her lowest points, writing to Overman, "I feel very well I guess at times I feel like I just can't stay here any longer though. I wish I could get well enough to leave here for at least a little while. I guess I'm just tired of Sanatarium life." She had not been able to walk on her own for some time. She apologized for all the trouble Overman was going through to try to get special shoes to help her walk, adding, "I've waited so long to walk I feel like a little longer won't matter."[103]

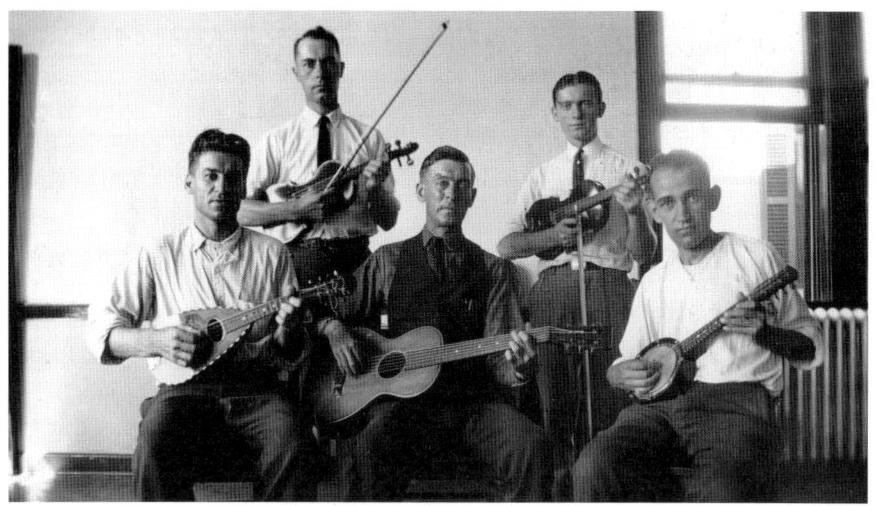

A string band at Waverly Hills Sanatorium made up of patients and employees, circa early 1920s. In 1929, Stella Hatfield took up playing the ukulele to help pass the time. *Edward Arthur Waverly Hills Photograph Collection, 019PC9.10, Filson Historical Society.*

Hatfield's troubles with her hip and limb continued through the fall of 1930, leading up to some of her most despondent letters. One was written on October 12 to her friend "Dearest Ruth" at Hazelwood Sanatorium, where Hatfield had evidently received treatment before her time at Waverly Hills. Hatfield told Ruth that she had been thinking of her and "the old gang" at Hazelwood. She expressed a feeling of despair about her current situation at Waverly Hills:

> *Sometimes I write letters to you all I never send because I read them over and they are so blue I wont send them. But I'm not going to read this one over at all. I'm so unhappy I could die at times. But how can I get away from here? I'm just tired of San*[atorium] *life I guess.*
>
> *And they are so strict on us over here can't speak to the boys without getting in trouble. I hate our doctor on this floor. I never speak to him unless I have to.*
>
> *And* [Dr.] *Miller isn't much better. I believe I would like to love doctor Turner to death if I could see him again. And I miss Mrs. Turner we have no one like her over here.*
>
> *There is only two ways to get out of here for me and that is get well or die. I feel like jumping off the roof, at times, but I guess I just haven't the nerve.*

And I'm so unhappy I can't get well. Most of the nurses are very good to us. But it is so lonely it's just like a grave yard on this fifth floor.[104]

The Turners referred to in the letter were Hazelwood superintendent Dr. Paul A. Turner and his wife and Hazelwood executive secretary, Alice Turner. The letter ended up in the hands of Alice Turner, who passed it on to Robert Bingham, telling him it was "written by little Stella Hatfield to one of the girls here at the Sanatorium which pitifully tells its own tale. Knowing your interest in her I feel that you should have this letter."[105]

Perhaps because of the October 12 letter, the Turners, Bingham, and Emily Overman all stepped up their efforts to help Stella Hatfield. Overman arranged for Hatfield to be taken into the city by a chauffeur several times to see Dr. William Barnett Owen, a nationally renowned orthopedic surgeon who had headed the medical staff at Louisville's Kosair Crippled Children Hospital since its founding in 1925. Dr. Owen examined and had an

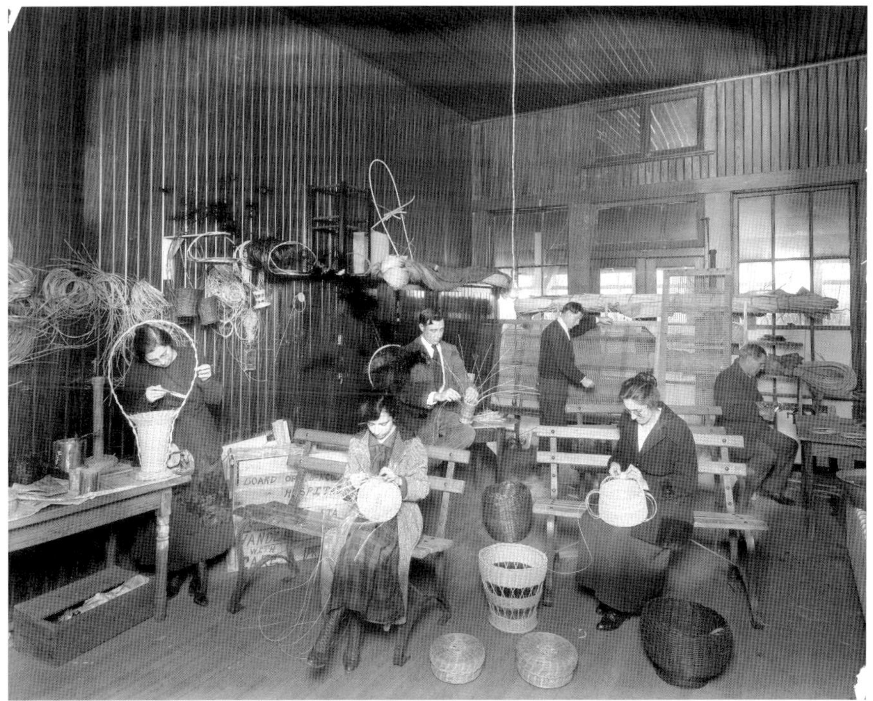

Patients making baskets in the main sanatorium's occupational therapy shop, 1926. Stella Hatfield wrote of working on sewing and painting projects at the "O.T. shop." *Caufield and Shook Collection, 40464, Archives and Special Collections, University of Louisville.*

X-ray made of the leg currently giving Hatfield trouble, and he planned to drain fluid from it. In Hatfield's final letter, dated November 28 after the Thanksgiving holiday, she apologized to Overman for having to make so many trips to go see Dr. Owen, "as it is so far out and so much expense to Mr. Bingham." The closing part of her letter expressed her gratitude:

> *But I want you and Mr. Bingham to know I do appreciate everything you have done for me. And I hope God will let me live and be able to do some good for someone.*
>
> *I had a real nice Thanksgiving. I went to Hazelwood Sanatorium for the day. Mrs. Turner came over and got me. She is Doctor Paul Turner's wife. Doctor and Mrs. Turner has been so good to me.*
>
> *In fact everyone here and everywhere is just Wonderful to me. I hope you had a nice Thanksgiving.*
>
> *I've been list*[en]*ing to the parade over the radio and I sure did enjoy it. We all did. I enjoy the radio so much always.*
>
> *I'll close thanking you and Mr. Bingham for everything.*[106]

Seven months later, on May 8, 1931, Stella Hatfield died at City Hospital, with the cause identified as tuberculosis of the hip with complications of early bronchopneumonia.[107] Her case of tuberculosis was a hard and harrowing one, and her life at Waverly Hills was extremely difficult for her to bear, even with the amenities and activities available to her at the main sanatorium. Yet she acknowledged the support offered to her and expressed the hope that, in turn, she would one day be able to leave and "do some good for someone."

Chapter 5

HELP DURING THE GREAT DEPRESSION

Following the stock market crash on October 24, 1929, the United States fell into a deepening economic crisis with growing rates of unemployment. Waverly Hills Sanatorium persevered through the Great Depression of the 1930s with the critical support of city and county funds, contributions from local organizations, and new federal government programs. High numbers of patients were admitted to Waverly Hills during the decade. In 1930, Waverly Hills Sanatorium had 242 employees and housed an average of 450 patients per day, and it was large enough to receive its own post office the following year. In 1937, the average number of patients per day had increased to around 500.[108]

In 1930, Dr. Benjamin L. Brock took over the head physician and superintendent position at Waverly Hills Sanatorium after Dr. Oscar Miller left the position. Dr. Miller retained his title as Waverly Hills medical director but focused on tuberculosis field and dispensary work in the city and county. The following year, the Board of Tuberculosis Hospital moved the Waverly Hills Tuberculosis Clinic to its new quarters at 235 East Chestnut Street. In 1934, the board claimed a significant amount of credit for a 60 percent drop in deaths from tuberculosis in the city and the county in the past twenty-three years: "The big decline has been due to natural causes, in part, but mainly due to the progressive work of the Waverly Hills Sanatorium and clinic."[109]

Waverly Hills received positive publicity for its facilities and patient care during the 1930s. In April 1934, the main sanatorium housed Kentucky governor Ruby Laffoon as a patient. Governor Laffoon did not suffer from tuberculosis but rather needed "rest" and "vacation" from his work in the capital. He spent nearly a week at the main sanatorium, declaring upon his release, "I never felt better in my whole life than I feel right now. They treated me fine down there. I feel like a new man."[110] Later in the 1930s, Waverly Hills was one of the sanatoriums featured by the National Tuberculosis Association in its educational film *On the Firing Line*. Prominent tuberculosis experts called Waverly Hills the leading sanatorium in the South and "one of the most outstanding in the country." A newspaper article in 1938 heralded Waverly Hills for its new "postural treatment," which it said Dr. Benjamin Brock and other medical staff had been working on for three years. The treatment consisted simply of having patients elevate their feet above their heads "to rest the lungs." Perhaps it was a cost-saving treatment to offer during financially precarious times.[111]

For their part, patients and their families during the Great Depression struggled not just with tuberculosis and institutional treatment but also with widespread unemployment. In a weekly *Courier-Journal* column titled "Along King's Highway" dating back to the 1920s, Linda Hope Carew presented pleas for help from local residents, including Waverly Hills patients. In 1930, a woman who identified herself as a widow with three children wrote that she and her nine-year-old son were patients at Waverly Hills. She asked for "two kimonos, two pairs of pajamas, and a pair of bedroom slippers size 5½" for herself and "some lightweight overalls and wash suits, and stockings, size 8" for her son. Women with husbands hospitalized at Waverly Hills asked for bedding, clothes, and food for family members still at home. Former patients asked for help getting a job, preferably one involving outdoor work.[112]

In 1932, "G.B." wrote a letter to the editor of the *Courier-Journal* outlining "the obstacles which we patients of the Waverly Hills Sanatorium face." A major problem was the enduring stigma of tuberculosis: "People who have relatives and beloved ones in the institution prefer keeping it as secret as possible to prevent their being handicapped in daily life, as many people go so far as to avoid coming into contact with anyone who has close relatives here." The aversion to tuberculosis patients extended to those who had been discharged from Waverly Hills as cured. They were "branded as tuberculars because they have had the courage to enter this institution and fight the hardest battle they have ever fought." It was almost impossible for former patients to find jobs, as employers were reluctant to hire someone who had been treated at the sanatorium. "This is unjust," the letter-writer noted, "because the purpose of this institution is to take the dangerous

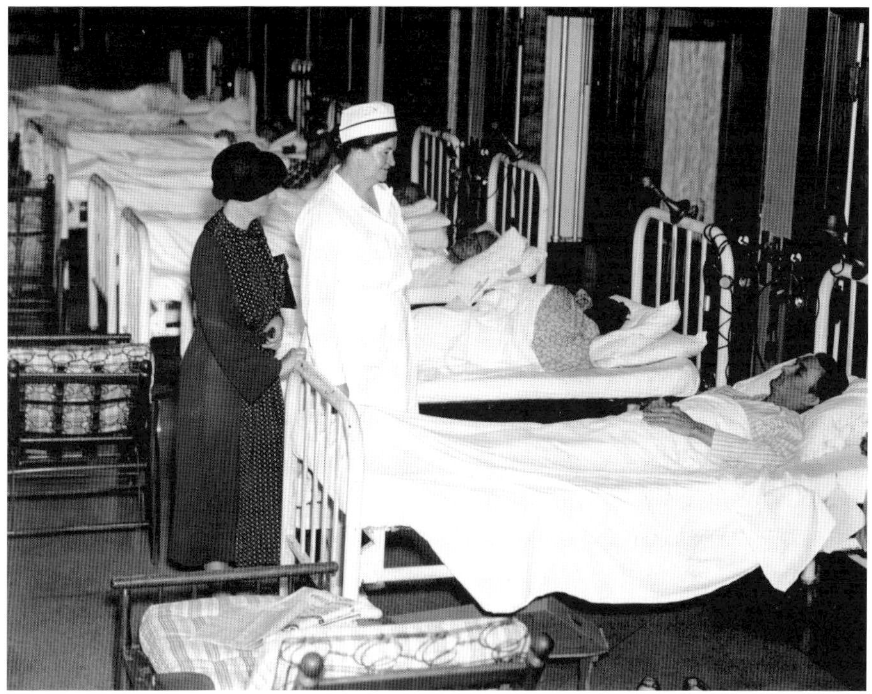

A woman and a nurse visiting male patients in their beds, 1936. *Courtesy of* Louisville Courier-Journal.

cases out of the society of the well people and when one is discharged from the institution as cured, there is absolutely no danger in his associating with others." The dangerous people, the letter concluded, are the ones who work in offices and factories, complain of their health, and "in many, many cases, really have tuberculosis" but refuse to seek treatment at the sanatorium. Patients who accepted treatment at Waverly Hills should be praised for helping to protect public health, the letter-writer argued, rather than seen as a perpetual threat.[113]

Due in part to the difficulties faced by parents diagnosed with tuberculosis, many children were admitted to Waverly Hills during the 1930s. Among the Waverly Hills patients appearing in the National Tuberculosis Association's *On the Firing Line* film was a group of white children identified as "children of tuberculosis parents who cannot be properly protected otherwise" and who are "cared for in a special department of the sanatorium."[114]

Tuberculosis case–finding programs contributed to the admission of children to Waverly Hills Sanatorium, including many with possible incipient or early cases. The Waverly Hills Tuberculosis Clinic worked with

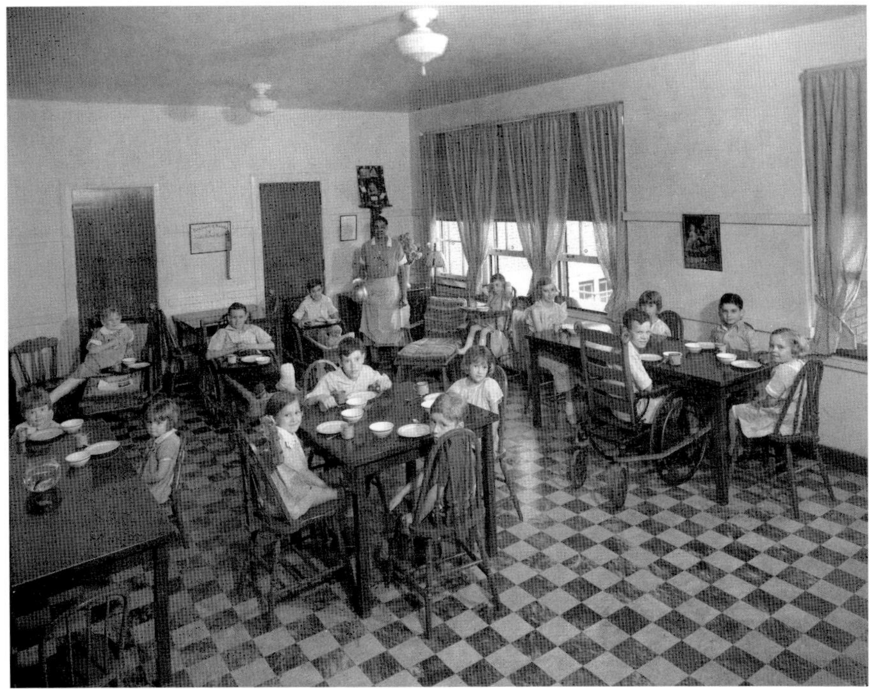

Children in the dining room at Waverly Hills, 1938. *Caufield and Shook Collection, 151959, Archives and Special Collections, University of Louisville.*

city and county health departments, the Louisville Tuberculosis Association, and local schools to expand screening of children and teenagers with the tuberculin skin test, a less cumbersome process than sputum tests and X-rays. If a child tested positive, a physician would follow up with an X-ray and likely a recommendation of sanatorium treatment. In December 1937, a portable X-ray machine was brought to Highland Junior High School to screen students for tuberculosis. The *Courier-Journal* article covering the event featured the headline "Students Hail X-Ray Test as Fun." According to one source, efforts to screen for tuberculosis among school-aged children during the 1930s identified roughly 50 percent with "some indication of the need for treatment."[115]

At the beginning of the 1930s, the Board of Tuberculosis Hospital lobbied the city and county for funds to build two new hospital units at Waverly Hills, one for children and one for Black patients. At this point, the Black hospital housed one hundred patients in "crowded and unsuitable quarters." Board president A.H. Bowman said a children's building was also a "pressing need," with eighty children currently housed in two old wood structures.[116]

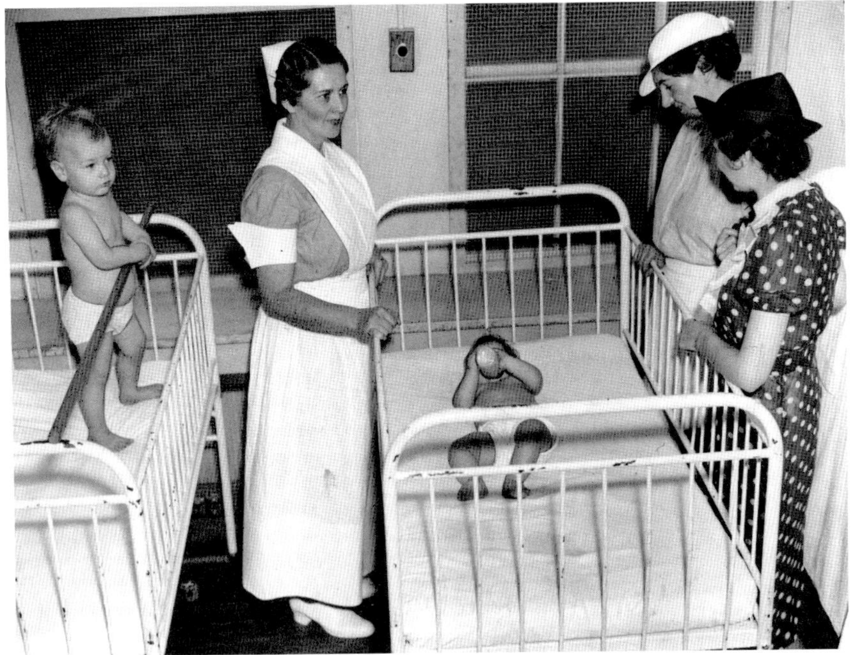

Nurse Florence Cook and two members of the Family Service Organization, Emma Mauer and M.A. Ruter, visit the Waverly Hills nursery, 1936. At the time, the nursery held eight babies ranging in age from one month to two years old. *Courtesy of* Louisville Courier-Journal.

Only one building was constructed—a brick unit that opened in 1933 and housed seventy-five Black patients by 1934. The facility was designed by D.X. Murphy and located near the older Black hospital, and both buildings housed Black patients. Originally, the new building was meant to house Black children. According to the *Louisville Leader*, members of the Waverly Hills committee of the City Federation of Colored Women had worked for four years with Waverly Hills nurse supervisor Esther Barrens, "giving cheer to the sick, and the new building for children is a climax to the committee's untiring efforts." Alice B. Crutcher, chair of the committee, organized a program on February 26, 1933, for the dedication of "the new building for children."[117] Several weeks later, a letter to the *Louisville Leader* lauded the "splendid new addition to the colored division at Waverley Hills" but noted that the building ended up being filled with adult bed patients instead of children. Despite the shift in who was housed in the new unit, the letter concluded with expressions of gratitude to those who had helped make it a reality, including "the staff of Waverly, the finest anywhere, with their kindly sympathy and cheerful help"; Dr. Ballard "for his faithfulness and

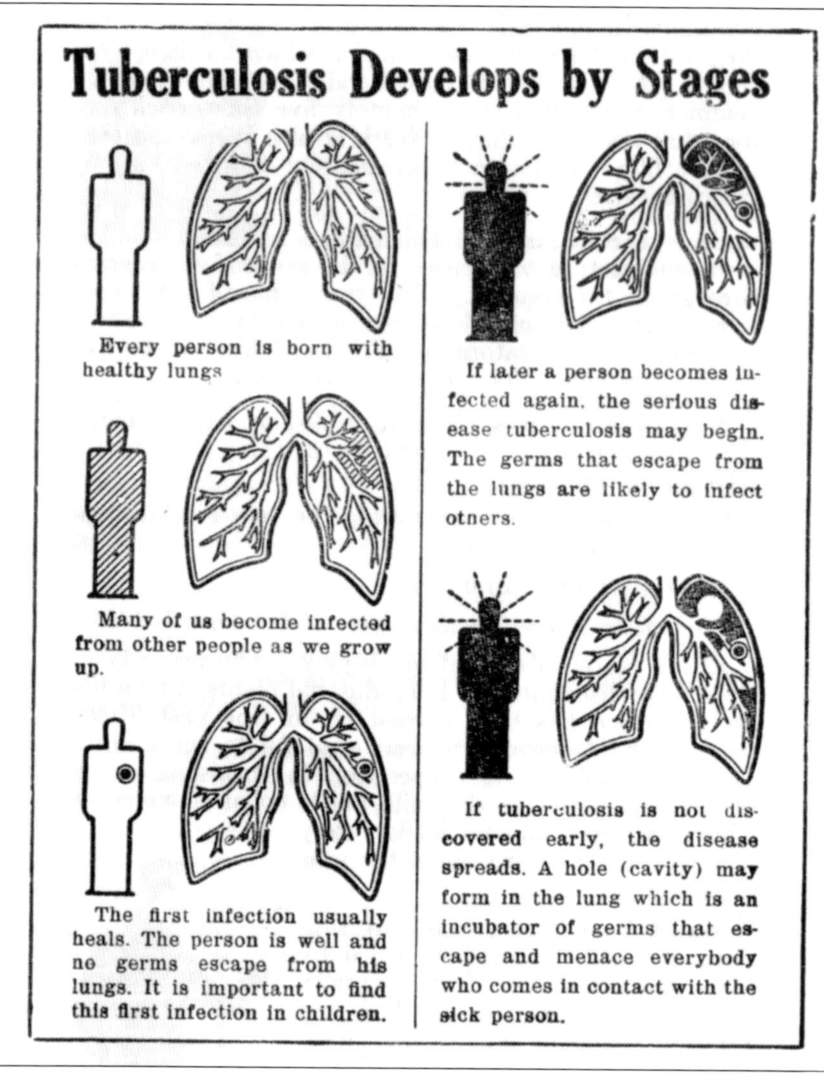

Tuberculosis Develops by Stages

Every person is born with healthy lungs

Many of us become infected from other people as we grow up.

The first infection usually heals. The person is well and no germs escape from his lungs. It is important to find this first infection in children.

If later a person becomes infected again, the serious disease tuberculosis may begin. The germs that escape from the lungs are likely to infect otners.

If tuberculosis is not discovered early, the disease spreads. A hole (cavity) may form in the lung which is an incubator of germs that escape and menace everybody who comes in contact with the sick person.

This graphic includes a sentence about the importance of catching the "first infection" of tuberculosis in children. 34th Annual Report of the Louisville Tuberculosis Association, *1938, pamphlet 614.542 L888, Filson Historical Society.*

earnestness in the work he has put before him and what he has done in the past"; and "Mrs. Barrens, supervisor, for her never tiring efforts to bring about the results that we now have to show."[118]

Esther Barrens served as an important liaison in the 1930s among Black patients at Waverly Hills, charitable associations in Louisville, and local and national health professionals. In Louisville, she was an active member of the Charity Pity Club and the Quinn Chapel African Methodist Episcopal Church. In 1933, Barrens organized a health program at the Quinn Chapel featuring talks by Dr. Ballard and other medical professionals. She helped plan "Negro Health Week" programs for the public at Waverly Hills throughout the decade. In August 1935, the *Louisville Leader* reported that she had "motored" down to New Orleans in her car with Dr. Ballard and Dr. John Nurse to attend a meeting of the National Association of Colored Nurses, Dentists and Physicians. Unlike Dr. Ballard, who lived with his family in a private home behind the Black hospital at Waverly Hills, Esther Barrens and her family lived in the city on West Madison Street. At her home in 1938, she hosted graduate nurses attending a meeting of the Southern Tuberculosis Conference and Southern Association of Sanatoriums in Louisville.[119]

Coordinating with Esther Barrens and other staff, many charitable associations from Louisville contributed to the comfort and care of Black patients at Waverly Hills. For Valentine's Day in 1929, the Buds of Promise Health and the Literary Club of the Booker T. Washington School donated boxes of candy to the nineteen Black children who were hospitalized at Waverly Hills. In December, the Phyllis Wheatley Branch of the Young Women's Christian Association brought candy and fruit to the hospital for the Christmas holiday. For Easter in April 1933, Alice Crutcher led the Waverly Hills committee of the City Federation of Colored Women in gathering donations for pajamas for patients from an impressively long list of local associations: the Charity Pity Club, Women's Improvement Club, Vocational Club, Lampton Aid Society, Mamie E. Steward Friendly Group, Chrysanthemum Club, Loyal Charity Club, Ladies Sewing Circle, Eta Zeta Sorority, Auxiliary of the Merciful Savior Church, Friendly Twelve, Home Beautiful, Missionary Club of Broadway Temple, Sisterhood of Zion Baptist Church, West End Gloom Chaser, Oak and Ivy Club, Chummy Club, and the Stitch and Chatter Club. Members of the Waverly Hills committee put a flower next to the bed of each patient and sponsored an egg hunt for children. The Charity Pity Club made garments for children, visited patients to "cheer hearts," and held parties to celebrate patients' birthdays. In December 1939, the Faithful Sewing Club donated fruit to and held devotional services for patients at the hospital.[120]

In addition to the assistance of local associations, New Deal federal government programs helped to support Waverly Hills Sanatorium during the Great Depression. The Waverly Hills administration and white-run associations in Louisville worked with the short-lived Civil Works

Administration (CWA) in 1933–34 and the longer-lasting Works Progress Administration (WPA) after 1935 to enhance services at the main sanatorium. In 1934, the Louisville Women's City Club spearheaded a CWA project to improve library services at Waverly Hills. The project hired two librarians and two typists to catalogue books at the main sanatorium library, and the staff took around a cart of books and magazines to patients in their beds. Magazine subscriptions were provided by local associations, including the Highland Mother's Club, Crescent Hill Women's Club, the local chapter of the National Council of Jewish Women, the Unitarian church, and the Shawnee Woman's Club.[121]

The WPA hired unemployed men from the city and county for a roadway and landscaping project and paid the salary of an adult education teacher at Waverly Hills. In 1937, Esther Haskell headed the adult education program, teaching classes in typing, shorthand, bookkeeping, spelling, and arithmetic. Haskell also put parties "under her jurisdiction," and a *Courier-Journal* article included images of some of the sixteen- and seventeen-year-old female patients who participated in a Halloween party on the "girls' wing" at the

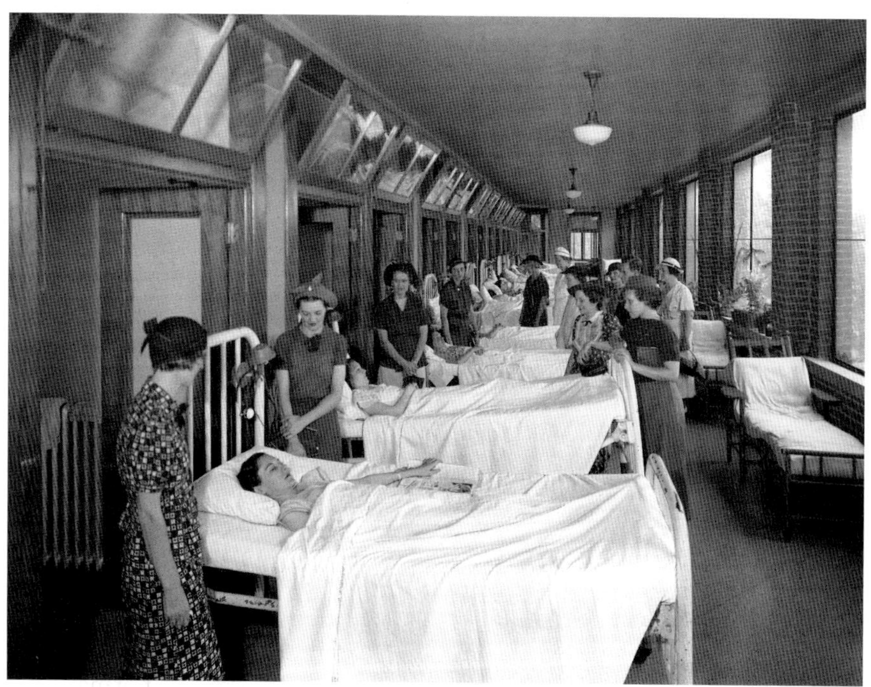

Clubwomen standing around female patients in beds on a sun porch of the main sanatorium, 1936. Herald-Post, *94.18.0758, Archives and Special Collections, University of Louisville.*

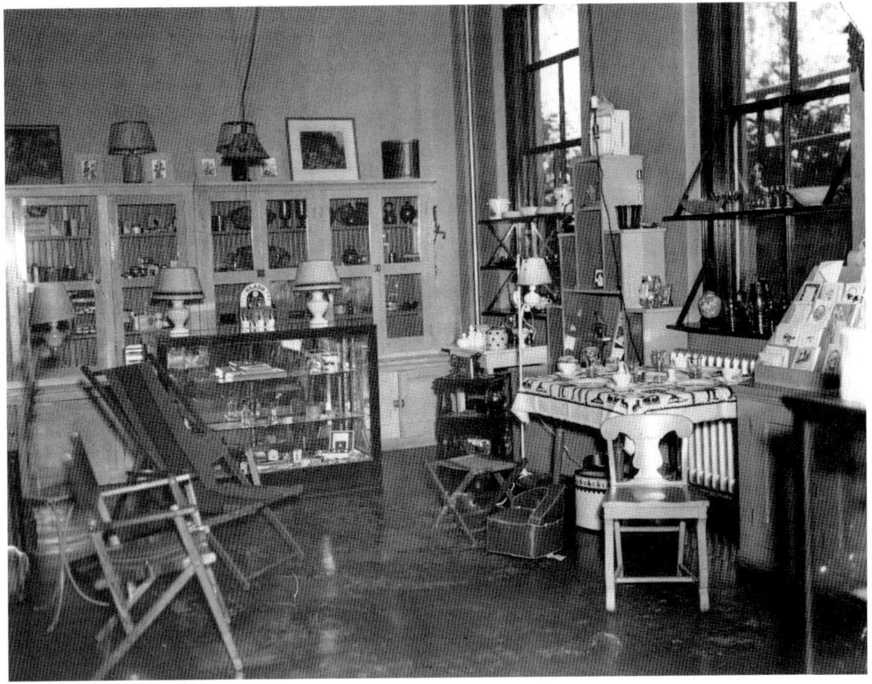

The Waverly Shop in the main sanatorium, 1935. The Women's Advisory Board ran the Waverly Shop to sell goods to patients and employees, with profits funding improvements and programs. *Courtesy of* Louisville Courier-Journal.

main sanatorium.[122] There is no indication whether these library services, education classes, or parties were made available to Black patients at Waverly Hills in the 1930s.

The Ohio River flood in early 1937 had a small impact on Waverly Hills Sanatorium compared to the widespread damage inflicted on other areas of Louisville and Jefferson County. The floodwaters did not reach Waverly Hills Sanatorium, but the high grounds of the main sanatorium served as an important refuge to nearby residents of Valley Station. Of the 1,500 individuals rescued from floodwaters and brought to Waverly Hills, 550 remained for four days in the main sanatorium's large recreation rooms. One of the refugees, Eugenia Hinderer, gave birth to a boy, reported to be the first obstetrical case in the history of the main sanatorium. In reference to the flood refugees who received shelter and food at Waverly Hills, the *Courier-Journal* noted, "They fared well, since the sanatorium's patients normally eat chicken, eggs, and the best of meat and vegetables."[123]

Chapter 6

WARTIME CHANGES AND POSTWAR CHALLENGES

The outbreak of World War II, with the United States entering the war in December 1941, launched a new era for Waverly Hills Sanatorium. Once again, military camps became breeding grounds for tuberculosis. Wartime industrial jobs accelerated the migration of rural residents to urban areas, where congested factory floors and crowded housing conditions posed renewed challenges to the control of infectious diseases. In 1942, Louisville health officials reported a "decided rise" in local cases of tuberculosis and syphilis. Due to people joining the military or working for higher wages in other wartime industries, Waverly Hills operated on a "skeleton medical staff" during much of the war. Staff shortages continued in the postwar period through the 1950s.[124]

Early in the war, Waverly Hills Sanatorium underwent a critical shift in management. Since Waverly Hills was a public institution supported by city and county taxes, many officials had long believed it should be managed by a public agency rather than by the independent Board of Tuberculosis Hospital. Beginning with the establishment of the Board of Tuberculosis Hospital by the Kentucky legislature in 1906, members had been appointed by the Louisville mayor and reported to no government entity. In early 1942, a proposed merger of the Louisville Department of Health and Jefferson County Board of Health was put before the Kentucky state legislature for approval. The merger included a plan to put both Louisville's City Hospital and Waverly Hills Sanatorium under the control of the consolidated City-County Board of Health.

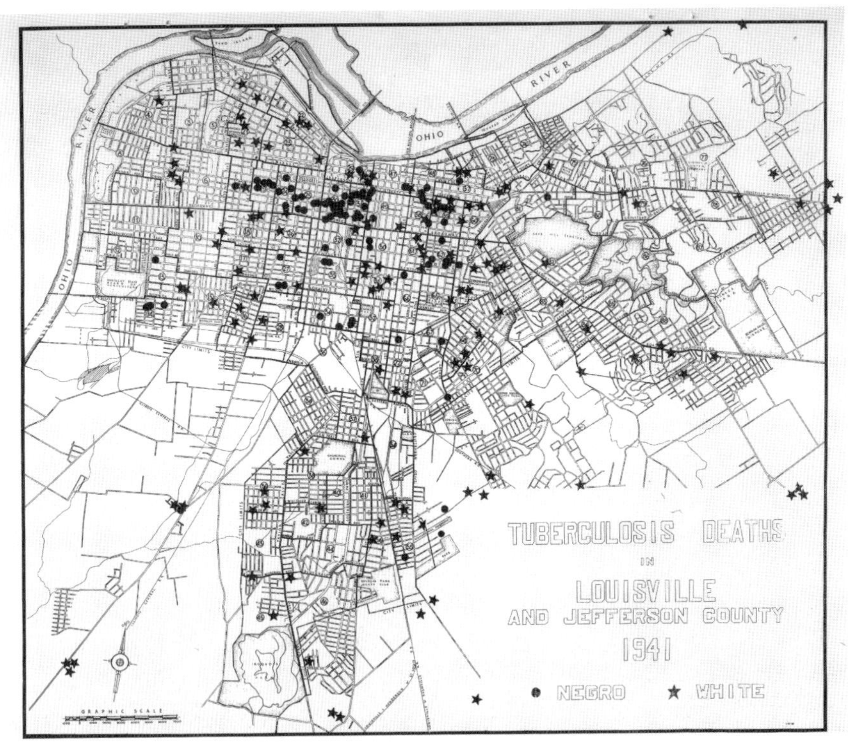

A map showing locations of deaths from tuberculosis in Louisville among Black and white residents, 1941. *"Tuberculosis in Louisville," Report of the Tuberculosis Committee of the Health Council, December 1942, Kornhauser Health Sciences Library, University of Louisville.*

Most vocal in their opposition to the proposal were Board of Tuberculosis Hospital member Edward Hilliard and Waverly Hills medical director Dr. Oscar Miller, who believed the sanatorium needed to remain independent of political influence and intervention. They said Waverly Hills should not fall prey to what they claimed was the local government's mismanagement of City Hospital. With the debate over the merger occurring during World War II, Hilliard's testimony to the Kentucky Senate compared Waverly Hills to "one of those little European countries which was getting along all right until somebody began shoving." Hilliard, who had suffered from tuberculosis as a child, took out a full-page advertisement in the *Louisville Times*, imploring readers to "Help Save Waverley!" and asking, "Do you want Waverley and the City Hospital under the same management?" A Louisville resident, Lila Rayner, invoked similar concerns in a letter to the *Courier-Journal*: "Waverley Hills is so far ahead of the other institutions in Kentucky that it would be criminal to change it."[125]

LOUISVILLE HEALTH DEPARTMENT

LEADING CAUSES OF DEATH

1938, 1939, 1940

NUMERICAL ORDER FOR EACH YEAR			NAME OF DISEASE	NUMBER OF DEATHS FOR EACH YEAR			RATES FOR EACH YEAR		
1938	1939	1940		1938	1939	1940	1938	1939	1940
1	1	1	HEART DISEASE	1004	1155	1183	316.9	363.3	370.9
2	2	2	CEREBRAL HEMORRHAGE	408	400	388	128.8	125.8	121.6
3	3	3	CANCER	347	356	385	109.5	112.0	120.2
4	5	4	NEPHRITIS, ALL FORMS	281	238	294	88.7	74.9	92.2
5	4	5	PNEUMONIA, ALL FORMS	251	270	205	79.2	84.9	63.9
7	7	6	DISEASES OF EARLY INFANCY	147	159	195	46.4	50.0	61.2
6	6	7	TUBERCULOSIS, ALL FORMS	213	192	191	67.2	60.4	59.9
8	8	8	ARTERIOSCLEROSIS	97	103	96	90.6	32.4	30.1
		9	AUTOMOBILE ACCIDENTS			90			28.2
9	9	10	DIABETES	70	70	78	22.1	22.0	24.5
	10	11	INFLUENZA		68	78		21.4	24.5
10			DIARRHEA AND ENTERITIS (UNDER 2 YEARS)	61			19.3		
			VIOLENT & ACCIDENTAL DEATHS	294	286	335	92.8	90.0	105.0

The leading causes of death in Louisville in 1938–40. Tuberculosis had fallen from the number-one cause of death in 1900 to number seven in 1940. *Louisville Health Department, 1940 annual report, Filson Historical Society.*

Leading the fight for putting Waverly Hills Sanatorium under the management of a consolidated Board of Health were Louisville mayor Wilson W. Wyatt and Dr. Hugh R. Leavell, the head officer of the Louisville Department of Health. Mayor Wyatt did not mince words in characterizing opponents of consolidation as irrational. "I am not impressed," he said, "by the unreasoning and emotional opposition to this program because of sentimental attachment to one disease." Dr. Leavell pointed out that for every city resident who died from tuberculosis, twenty-two died from other causes. He and others identified the independent Board of Tuberculosis Hospital as an "outmoded form of management" with access to a disproportionate amount of taxes. The board lacked supervision from any public administrative department, and the sanatorium was supported "in perpetuity" by city and county tax levies. With changing conditions and growing threats from other diseases, "the institution may outlive its usefulness."[126]

Supporters of the consolidation drew attention to Waverly Hills's significant budget in comparison to the "greatly undernourished" finances of City Hospital. Waverly Hills had a budget of $425,000, with allocations of around $291,000 from the city and $134,000 from the county in 1940. City Hospital, which was characterized as "understaffed" and "deficient in needed supplies," operated on an allocation of $517,122 from the city in 1940. Waverly Hills, treating one disease, received four-fifths of what City Hospital was allotted to "care for a cross-section of the medical needs of a large city." As advocates for the health merger made clear, they did not want the quality of care at Waverly Hill to decline. Rather, redistribution of public funds meant standards would be raised for the underfinanced City Hospital.[127]

The state legislature approved the merger at the end of January 1942. The new Board of Health took over the management of Waverly Hills Sanatorium, the City Hospital, and public health work for the city and county. At its first meeting in March 1942, the Board of Health changed the name of City Hospital to Louisville General Hospital (decades later, the name would change to University Hospital when University of Louisville took ownership of the hospital in 1979).[128] In March 1945, the board implemented a change in the official spelling of Waverly Hills Sanatorium. The *Courier-Journal* outlined the variations of the sanatorium's name over time:

> *The Louisville and Jefferson County Board of Health has changed the spelling of the name of the tuberculosis sanatorium at Waverly Hills to make it conform with the spelling of the name of the post office there. This is the third official spelling the sanatorium's name has had.*
>
> *Originally the sanatorium was WAVERLY HILL SANATORIUM—only one "E" in the first word and no "S" in the second.*
>
> *Later the Board of Tuberculosis Hospital changed the name to WAVERLEY HILLS SANATORIUM—with "E" twice in the first word and an "S" added to the second.*
>
> *Now it's WAVERLY HILLS SANATORIUM—back to one "E" in the first word but retaining the "S" on the second.*[129]

The Board of Health quickly took up the work of increasing the number of beds for Black patients at Waverly Hills. In the summer of 1942, the Board of Health hired D.X. Murphy to design a two-story brick addition to

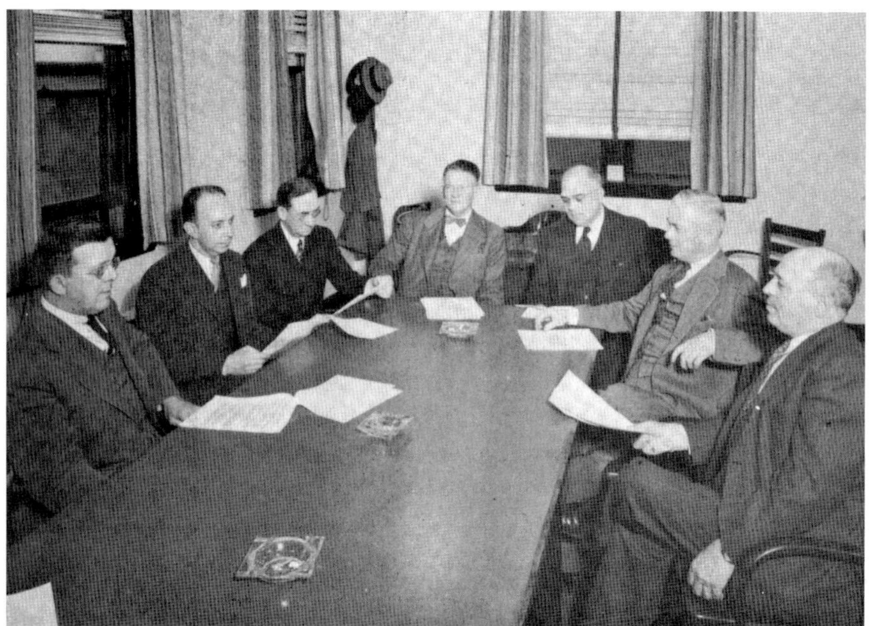

Members of the Louisville–Jefferson County Board of Health several years after the newly consolidated entity took over management of Waverly Hills Sanatorium in 1942. *Louisville–Jefferson County Board of Health, 1945 annual report, Kornhauser Health Sciences Library, University of Louisville.*

the brick Black hospital unit that opened in 1933, with new surgical facilities and 95 more beds to help expand what Dr. Orville Ballard described as an "overcrowded 116-bed capacity" in the current buildings. After the new addition opened in the fall of 1943, the Board of Health said Waverly Hills was providing "adequate facilities for Negro tuberculosis patients for the first time." However, only 35 beds in the new addition were available to patients at this point. The other 60 beds were in rooms not yet fully equipped, and the new surgical space was not expected to be ready until 1945. One of the buildings formerly used for Black patients, the thirty-year-old wood frame structure considered a fire hazard since the late 1910s, was repurposed for the housing of Black employees.[130]

Dr. Orville Ballard remained head of the Black hospital and received accolades both for his local work at Waverly Hills Sanatorium and for his national work giving talks around the country for the National Tuberculosis Association. Dr. Ballard recalled that when he took charge of the Black division at Waverly Hills in 1928, there were beds for only twenty-five patients. He expressed appreciation for the addition and for his years at

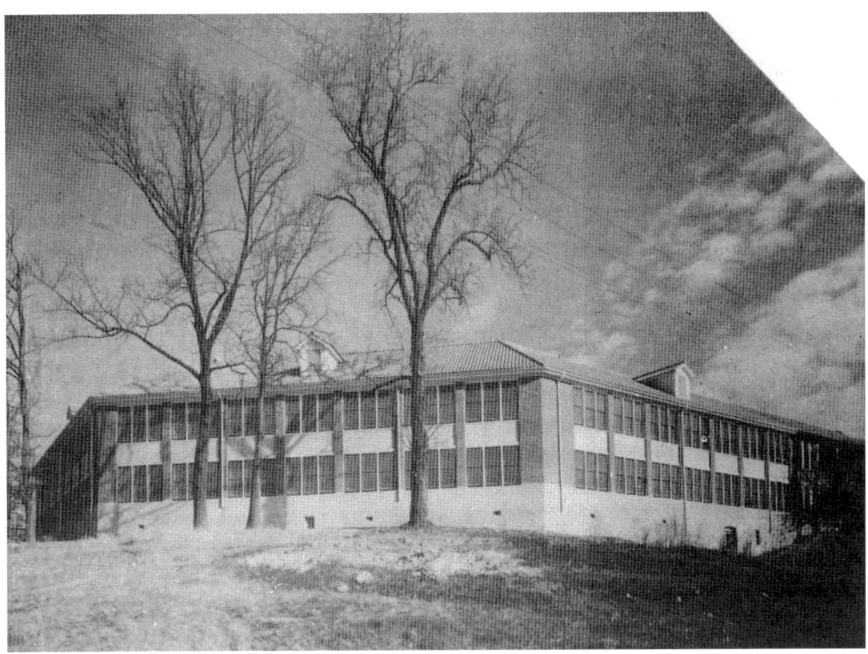

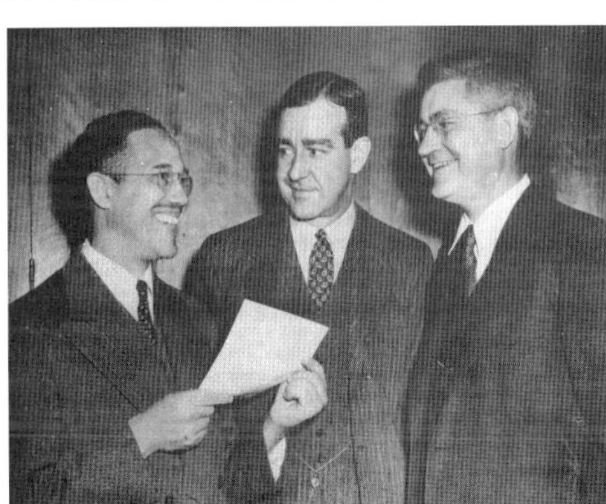

This page: Dr. Orville Ballard, Dr. Hugh Leavell, Dr. Benjamin Brock, and the new addition to the Black hospital at Waverly Hills Sanatorium. *Louisville–Jefferson County Board of Health, 1943 annual report, Kornhauser Health Sciences Library, University of Louisville.*

Waverly Hills Sanatorium. "I have always enjoyed the full privileges of a staff member here," he said, "and that has been a great help in my work." He said Waverly Hills was one of the first sanatoriums in the South to make pneumothorax therapy available to Black patients on a large scale. The same year the addition opened, Dr. Ballard was among three honored with the first annual award for distinguished postgraduate achievement by his alma mater, Howard University. The *Louisville Leader* noted how under Dr. Ballard's supervision, the Black division at Waverly Hills had made "remarkable gains."[131]

CHARGES OF BETTING AND DRINKING

In July 1945, S.A. Ruskjer, a former administrator of hospitals in the Kentucky towns of Paducah and Murray, succeeded W.R. Livermore as superintendent of Waverly Hills Sanatorium. He would remain in the position until the closure of Waverly Hills in 1961.[132] Ruskjer's first public battle as Waverly Hills superintendent was fought against Jefferson County commissioner E.P. White Jr. In September 1945, White accused the Waverly Hills administration of allowing betting and drinking among patients and staff, providing bad food, and pressuring employees to vote for Democratic candidates (White was a Republican), among other charges. Citing unnamed sources, White listed his accusations in a letter to the Board of Health and claimed the sanatorium was "slovenly, indifferently and partisanly operated."[133]

Some individuals defended Waverly Hills by saying the betting was small stakes and "therapeutic." A former patient explained how the illegal betting operated at Waverly Hills. First an orderly and later a succession of patients ran the handbook and the bets, which ranged from ten cents to a dollar on horse races. During the daily rest period from 1:00 to 3:00 p.m., when sanatorium rules mandated turning off radios, some patients turned the volume very low to track their bets. The bookie or his runner paid the winners the next morning, "and there never were any complaints" other than one argument over a three-way parlay. According to the former patient, betting was an activity well suited for bed-bound patients: "Lying there all day with nothing to do, it gives you some entertainment to bet on the horses and it isn't harming anybody." A former physician at the sanatorium agreed. "Up to 10 cents I would say the betting was beneficial for the patients," said the doctor, who asked the *Courier-Journal* to withhold his name.[134]

S.A. Ruskjer told the *Courier-Journal* and the Board of Health that he had already addressed the issues of drinking and betting since taking on the superintendent position in July. On his second day at Waverly Hills, he had found whiskey bottles lying around the grounds. After calling a meeting and telling the staff that no drinking on the job was allowed, he claimed he had not found any evidence of liquor on the premises. Regarding the accusations of betting, Ruskjer said an orderly, Louis Stone, had been admonished for taking small bets, had agreed to stop, and was still working part time at the sanatorium.[135]

Ruskjer denied the rest of the charges. To White's charge that "drinking by some of the favored patients who regularly visit Louisville and come back drunk is a common practice," Ruskjer insisted there were no privileged patients at Waverly Hills. But when patients left the sanatorium on a pass and came back under the influence of liquor (which he admitted happened "occasionally," most recently with a "Mr. Garland Pittard"), there was nothing the sanatorium could do to punish those individuals other than to discharge them. Kicking them out of the sanatorium would put a person with an active case of tuberculosis back in contact with the public. Only the passage of laws to "retain recalcitrant patients or chronic offenders" would authorize Waverly Hills to prohibit certain patients from leaving the institution. Ruskjer held there was nothing to substantiate White's accusation that orderlies at Waverly Hills "loaf around the woods and grounds, leaving the beds unmade for days." In response to White's charges claiming nurses at the sanatorium had been pressured to vote for Democratic candidates, Ruskjer said the nurses testified that the accusation was false.[136]

When the controversy over the charges continued, the Board of Health asked the Jefferson County Medical Society to investigate conditions at Waverly Hills. The report, issued in November, substantiated what had been said by Ruskjer. The committee concluded, "Waverly Hills Sanatorium is conducted in a skillful, efficient and economical manner by a well trained professional and business staff," with "high morale" among patients. The chief housekeeper, Ann Hollis, had been employed at Waverly Hills for more than thirty years, and both the white and the Black divisions of the sanatorium were found to uphold a standard of cleanliness. Patients were encouraged to take second helpings at their meals, and "food is served in heated containers in a manner comparable with that found in our best downtown cafeterias." The committee said the 15 percent of patients who left Waverly Hills against medical advice in recent years compared favorably with the average of 30 percent at tuberculosis sanatoriums nationwide.[137]

Others stepped forward to defend Waverly Hills. A *Courier-Journal* editorial criticized White for publicizing his charges before investigating them. Virginia Benham, an employee at Waverly Hills, wrote a letter to the *Courier-Journal* to testify to its cleanliness and ample amount of food. "We have to substitute eggs for breakfast on account of the meat shortage," she wrote, "but we can always go back for more if we don't have enough the first serving." She said she had voted Republican her entire adult life but now she would vote the Democratic ticket. A member of the Waverly Hills Women's Advisory Board claimed she visited over three hundred patients and heard only six complaints, which were "minor." A grand jury charged with carrying out inspections of public institutions said about Waverly Hills,

"The buildings are exceptionally clean, meals well prepared and excellently served, and workers and patients are well-treated."[138]

White continued his criticisms, but the Board of Health found little substance in his accusations and gave a unanimous vote of confidence to the Waverly Hills staff in the beginning of 1946. A letter to the *Courier-Journal* a few years later in 1948 offered the perspective of a current patient on the critiques leveled at the sanatorium. Samuel Long wrote:

> *I have been a patient at Waverly Hills for 14 months. During that time I have heard a lot of criticism about the food and the care the patients get. I have been in five hospitals in the last few years, and I was never treated better than I have been treated here. I am a steamboat fireman, and these people have been so nice to me I have forgotten how to cuss.*[139]

THE HOGS AND THE FARM

Late in the summer of 1945, before White launched his accusations at the Waverly Hills administration, one of S.A. Ruskjer's first major actions as superintendent was to ramp up the hog-breeding program. Employees enlarged the fenced-in area and the feeding platforms for the hogs. Lacking the facilities to butcher on site, process the meat, and have it government-inspected, the sanatorium sold the hogs to butchers in the city. "In all probability we buy back many of the hogs we have raised here," Ruskjer said. During a widespread meat shortage in 1946, Ruskjer expressed appreciation to Louisville meatpackers who tried to make sure the sanatorium had an adequate supply of pork: "Meat means the difference between life and death for tuberculosis patients."[140]

The hogs were lauded as "the pride of the Waverly Hills farm," with low costs and high profits. In 1949, the sale of more than 160 hogs brought in $10,000, with the number of hogs sold and the profits increasing in subsequent years. The hogs were fed food scraps and garbage from both Waverly Hills Sanatorium and General Hospital and then switched to a diet of corn from the farm at Waverly Hills a few weeks before they were old enough to sell at six months. In 1952, Waverly Hills installed garbage-cooking equipment as a sanitary step recommended by the State Department of Health.[141]

Like the Waverly Hills hogs, the farm helped the administration to deal with rising food prices in the post–World War II years. In 1945, the Board of Health approved investment in new farm equipment, including a tractor, and sold one of the two teams of mules used at Waverly Hills. The amount of land under cultivation doubled to eighty acres within a few years, producing crops of potatoes, onions, radishes, lettuce, squash, apples, corn, cabbage, cucumbers, green beans, and tomatoes.[142]

Updated kitchen equipment helped with the processing of produce into meals for patients. In 1946, the main sanatorium obtained five new ranges, two "deep fat fryolators," a five-compartment vegetable steamer, and a hood "that will take all fumes, food smells, gases, smoke and steam out of the kitchen." Writing of the sanatorium's "experienced chefs under the direction of efficient dietitians" who planned "scientifically balanced meals for each patient daily," the Board of Health put a modern spin on the long-held faith in wholesome food as a treatment for tuberculosis patients.[143]

TIGHT BUDGETS AND STAFF SHORTAGES

The hogs and the farm helped Waverly Hills administrators deal with the rising costs of hospital care in the post–World War II years. The financial burden of running both Waverly Hills Sanatorium and General Hospital and overseeing public health programs began to far exceed the city and county funds allotted to the health department. In early 1948, County Judge Horace M. Baker said the $650,000 spent annually on Waverly Hills—one-fourth of the health department's budget—was desperately needed for other public health work. Other members of the Board of Health agreed, saying the high cost of tuberculosis care was "perhaps their biggest problem" but pledging their support for the institution.[144]

In June 1946, the Board of Health announced a significant cut in funds and services for Waverly Hills Sanatorium and General Hospital, forcing both institutions to shut down several wings and discharge patients. Waverly Hills was expected to lower its capacity to 400 beds, discharging 50 to 75 patients even though "the cure may not be completed." Three wards at Waverly Hills—two pavilions and the partial fifth floor of the main sanatorium—were closed in July. This lowered the number of beds for white patients to 290 and kept the number of beds for Black patients at 110.[145]

To help deal with the budget cuts, the Board of Health instituted a new pay policy for patients at Waverly Hills to take effect on October 1, 1946. The board approved a graduated pay scale of one to four dollars a day, depending on what a patient could pay. Registrars from General

Hospital's admitting department would investigate each Waverly Hills patient's financial resources and family obligations, as they did with General Hospital patients.[146]

The graduated pay scale was the Board of Health's attempt to take part in several different models of health care at midcentury. One standard was Waverly Hills as a free institution for all patients. Another model was practiced by many private and public hospitals, which required patients of means to pay for their treatment but also provided charity wards for cash-poor patients. Then there was the newer system of private or employee-provided hospital insurance that emerged during the Great Depression, took hold during World War II, and expanded in the postwar years. As officials explained, if Waverly Hills Sanatorium gave up its status as a "free institution," it would be able to collect insurance payments for patients who had health insurance and federal government funds for patients who were veterans. For patients who did not have health insurance, Waverly Hills would collect what they were able to pay. For patients who lacked financial means, the sanatorium would continue to provide free board and treatment.[147]

In an opinion piece published in the *Courier-Journal* in August 1946, Louisville resident W.W. McCann argued vehemently that Waverly Hills Sanatorium should remain a free public institution. Drawing on the language of the Fifteenth Amendment of the United States Constitution, he said the Kentucky legislature had never intended Waverly Hills Sanatorium "to be anything but a free hospital for rich and poor, regardless of race, religion or previous condition of servitude." He also emphasized the rights of local taxpayers over the authority of the Board of Health and health department director Dr. John J. Phair to implement a change in the status of Waverly Hills as a free institution. "Wake up, taxpayers of Louisville," he wrote. "You pay City and County taxes for the support of Waverly Hills Tuberculosis Sanatorium. What right has the Louisville and Jefferson County Board of Health and Dr. John J. Phair to try to charge patients for treatments starting October 1?"[148]

Administrators implemented the new pay scale for Waverly Hills Sanatorium in October 1946, and early results showed almost 70 of the 380 patients at Waverly Hills able to pay something for their hospitalization. Most could only pay one dollar a day, the lowest amount on the scale, but one patient was found who could pay the maximum four dollars a day.[149] By 1950, however, many Waverly Hills patients were flat out refusing to pay for treatment. They claimed they had already paid in taxes, or they falsified their ability to pay. Some consulted lawyers who told them the sanatorium could not legally collect fees. Even one insurance company refused to pay, arguing that Waverly Hills was a government institution.[150]

Waverly Hills superintendent S.A. Ruskjer said local residents had long claimed a stake to the fruits—sometimes literally—of the sanatorium and its grounds. "When I first came here," he said, "people helped themselves to the fruit in our orchards, took our tomatoes, and even took full truckloads of water from here. When we told them to stop, they said they were taxpayers and were entitled to the produce because the institution is tax supported." In later years, the sanatorium would put up protective fences and "No Trespassing" signs around both the orchard and the sewage disposal area to try to keep people out.[151]

Along with rising costs and tight budgets, Waverly Hills dealt with ongoing staff shortages during the 1940s and 1950s. Dr. Benjamin Brock, the head physician at Waverly Hills since 1931, left in early 1946 to take a higher-paid federal position at Louisville's new Veterans Administration Hospital. He was replaced by Dr. Alvin B. Mullen, who had joined the medical staff of Waverly Hills in 1926 and had just returned to the sanatorium after a three-and-a-half-year stint in the armed forces. At the close of the 1940s, there were five vacancies on the medical staff. Dr. Mullen pointed to the "marked loss of interest" of physicians in openings at Waverly Hills when they were informed about the salary scale. To fill some of these positions, Waverly Hills began to hire physicians from other countries. One of them, Dr. Elmars Spunde, escaped with his wife, a laboratory technician, and their children from the Eastern Bloc country of Latvia and came to Waverly Hills to work after the end of World War II.[152]

In 1947, the Board of Health solidified an arrangement with Meharry Medical College, a historically Black medical school in Nashville, Tennessee, to send a resident physician and medical students to the Black hospital at Waverly Hills on a regular basis. According to Dr. Orville Ballard, the program would help alleviate not just the shortage of physicians at Waverly Hills but also in Louisville, which at this point had only about twenty-five Black physicians. "We hope we can induce some of Meharry's students to establish their practice in Louisville when they finish school," he said. "There's a crying need for at least twice as many Negro doctors as are here now." He and other health leaders pointed to the continued lack of training and hospital positions available to Black physicians or nurses. Other than Waverly Hills Sanatorium and the private Black-run Red Cross Hospital in Louisville, no other local hospital provided positions for Black medical staff. Not until 1953 would Dr. Ballard and Dr. Grace M. Jones become

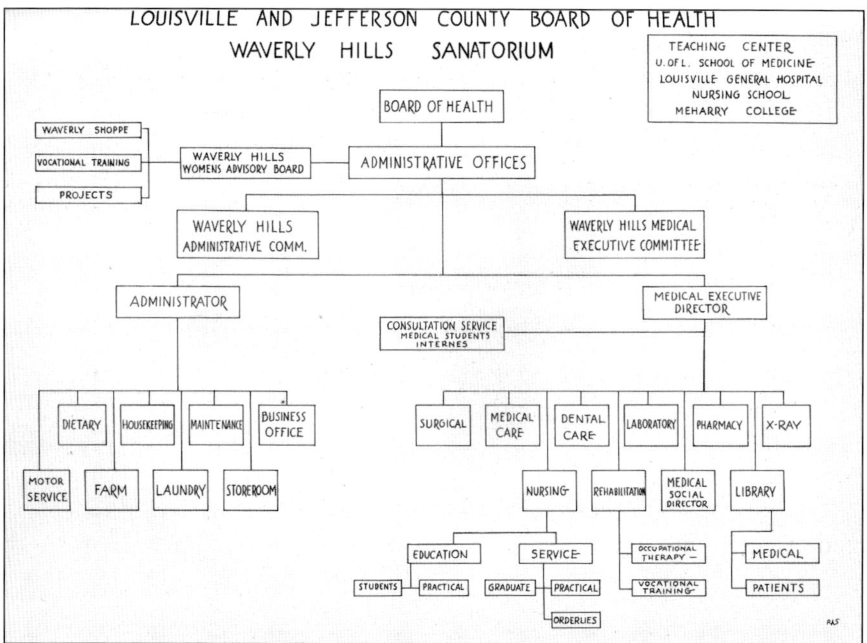

A chart showing the departmental structure of Waverly Hills Sanatorium in 1946. The box on the top right lists the schools and institutions affiliated with Waverly Hills. *Louisville–Jefferson County Board of Health, 1946 annual report, Kornhauser Health Sciences Library, University of Louisville.*

the first Black physicians to be appointed to the faculty of the University of Louisville Medical School.[153]

Waverly Hills administrators faced problems in hiring and retaining other employees as well, especially nurses and orderlies. They continued to hire many former patients, who were "carefully guarded against relapse from overwork." In 1954, Waverly Hills had 259 employees, with 200 of them living on the grounds, and there were some notable deaths and incidents among the staff that year. Just after midnight on May 26, forty-seven-year-old Mary Gladys Jones, a practical nurse, was killed when she was crossing Dixie Highway on foot after midnight and was hit by a car outside the entrance to Waverly Hills on Pages Lane. In August, longtime nurse supervisor Esther Barrens died at the age of sixty-six in her home in Louisville. In October, Robert Floyd, a twenty-nine-year-old former employee of Waverly Hills, was arrested on the grounds of the sanatorium and charged with "illegal possession of liquor on which taxes had not been paid." Pints and half pints of whiskey and gin had been confiscated from his car. He had worked in the kitchen at the main sanatorium until February

1953, at which point he quit and took a night shift at a distillery. He had been taking partly filled and rejected bottles of liquor at the distillery and selling them to employees at Waverly Hills until he was caught.[154]

A major incident earlier in 1954 involved the death of an employee at the hands of another employee. In March, fifty-one-year-old Edward Albert Bareis died after a fight with nineteen-year-old John Louis Griggs in the recreation room of a Waverly Hills building housing about thirty white male employees. At the murder trial, Griggs testified that Bareis was drunk and had "cursed and abused" him for an hour, heckling him for being a former convict recently released on parole from the Kentucky State Reformatory. Griggs said Bareis pulled out a knife and threatened to cut his guts out, but county police said they found no knife at the scene. Witnesses confirmed Bareis's verbal abuse of Griggs. They said Griggs had responded by hitting and kicking Bareis, who, according to physicians, died of a brain injury after suffering fractures of the skull, broken ribs, and a ruptured spleen. The jury was persuaded that Bareis had provoked the fight, and they acquitted Griggs of murder.[155]

Among the most pressing staffing issues needing attention in the 1950s were the old wooden structures serving as accommodations for many employees at Waverly Hills. The most "dilapidated and dangerous" was the hospital building dating from 1913 and used since 1943 for the housing of fifty Black employees. Beginning in 1954, plans were made to remodel the east wing of the two-story brick hospital for Black patients to house these employees and to move fifty Black female patients into a wing of the main sanatorium, where the white female wings had vacant beds. When the city and county delayed setting aside funds for the project, the *Courier-Journal* ran an article in early 1957 with images depicting the rusted bathroom facilities and holes in the ceiling and roof that let in water every time it rained. Black employees complained that a fifty-dollar charge for housing was automatically deducted from employees' paychecks, whether they lived at Waverly Hills or in Louisville, and no matter how substandard the accommodations allotted to them by the administration.[156]

Six months after the publication of the *Courier-Journal* article, the city allocated the $75,000 needed for the renovations. In 1958, Black female patients were transferred to a wing in the main sanatorium, evidently marking the first time Black patients obtained beds in that building. Approximately sixty male patients remained in the Black hospital. A third of the hospital building was converted into quarters for fifty Black employees. The renovation featured private bedrooms, a kitchen with stainless

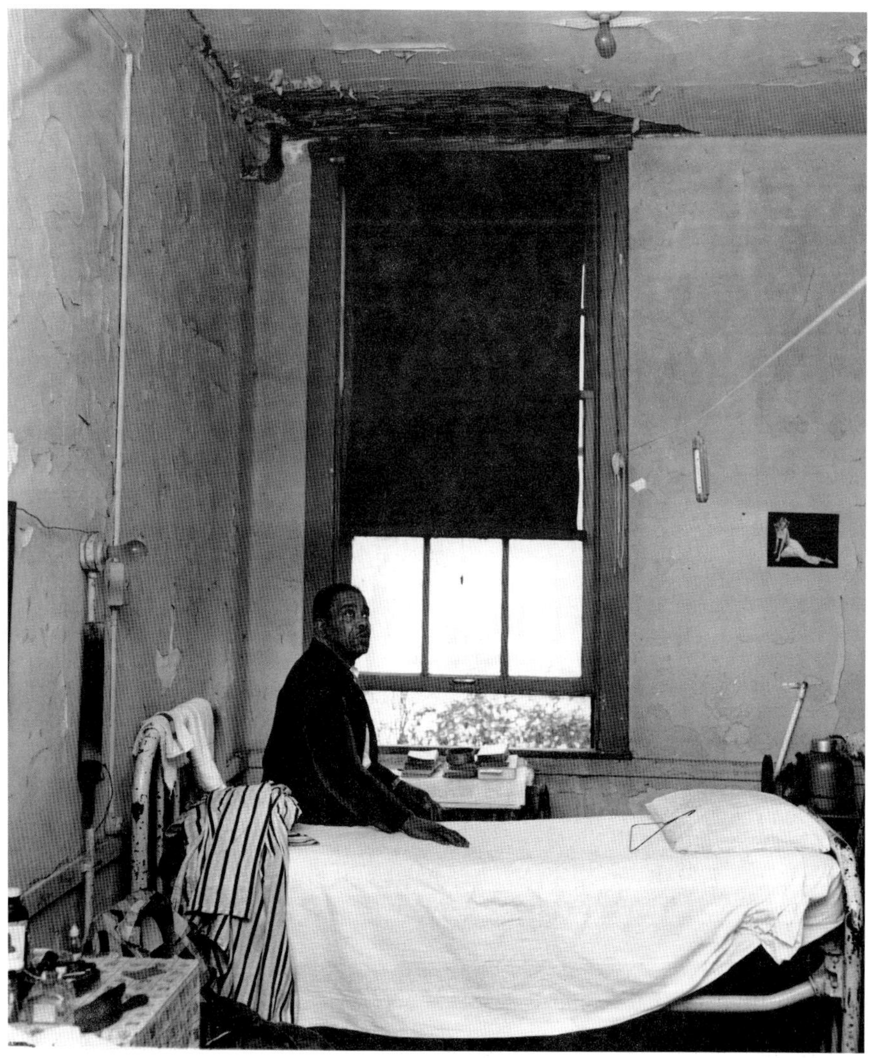

Above: Joseph Logan, an employee of Waverly Hills for twenty-two years, said his room in the building housing Black employees was "pretty bad," January 1957. *Courtesy of* Louisville Courier-Journal.

Opposite: Civil Service director Franklin H. Weir inspecting the run-down lavatory in the building housing Black employees, January 1957. *Courtesy of* Louisville Courier-Journal.

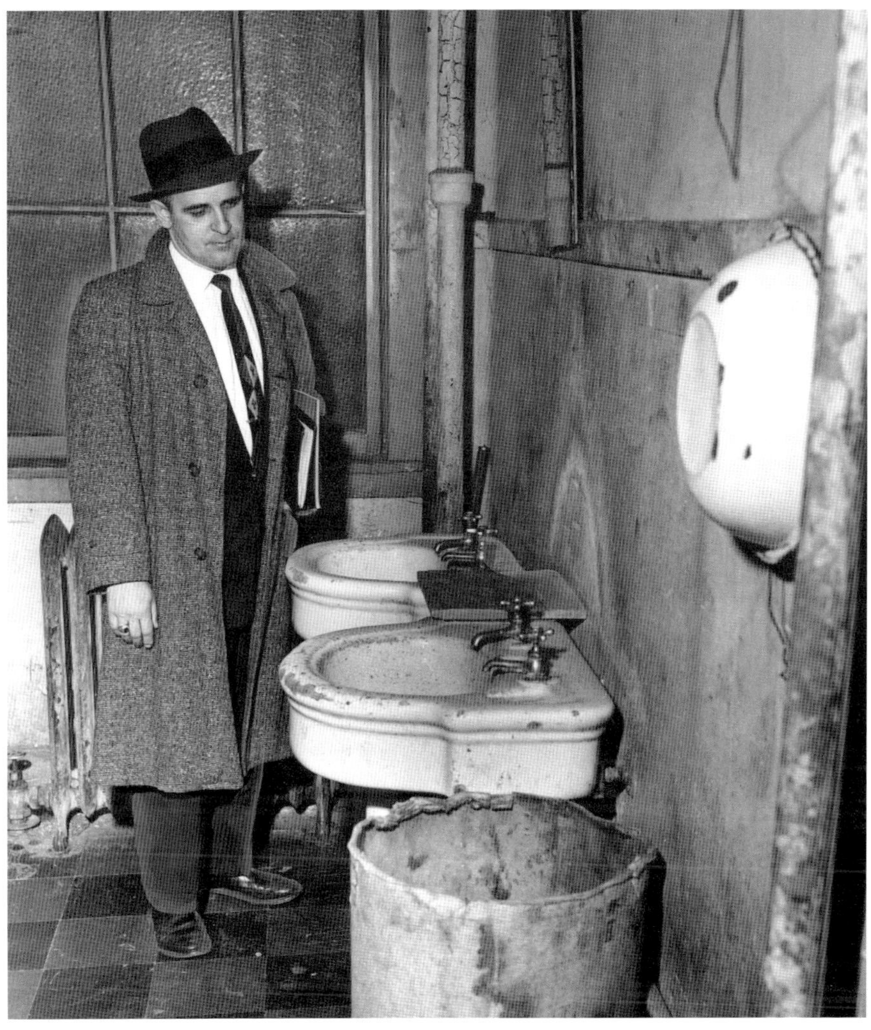

steel equipment, and a recreation area. The old building for employees, which had originally opened in 1913 as the hospital for advanced cases, was torn down.[157]

Asked about the new housing, nurse Lina Williams told the *Courier-Journal*, "I like it fine." After years of pushing for better housing, Black employees were not going to offer enthusiastic praise for what was so long in coming. Housekeeper Tillie Delaney said she had quit her job at Waverly Hills back in 1955. "I just couldn't stay in that old building," she said, and she went back to her home state of Tennessee after working at Waverly Hills for almost two decades. When she quit, she told Waverly Hills

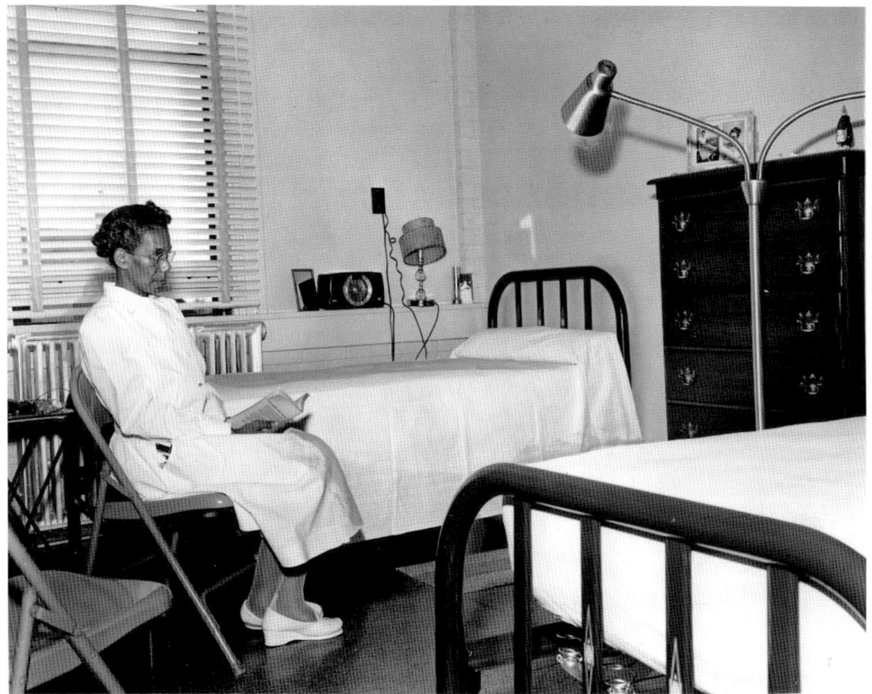

Nurse Lina Williams in her room in the newly renovated quarters for employees in a wing of the Black hospital, November 1958. She lived at Waverly Hills for five days of the week and also had a home in Louisville. *Courtesy of* Louisville Courier-Journal.

superintendent S.A. Ruskjer she would return only when Black employees received new quarters. When the new accommodations opened, she came back to Waverly Hills, and Ruskjer said morale had improved a great deal overall among the employees. It had been "all but impossible" to hire and retain Black employees until this point, he explained, and "we haven't lost any since we moved in here."[158]

Chapter 7

SANATORIUM LIFE AND NEW TREATMENTS AT MIDCENTURY

The years after World War II are often seen as a period of decline for tuberculosis sanatoriums, following the introduction of new antibiotics such as streptomycin. Waverly Hills, however, experienced fluctuations in its patient population, with decreases in the number of female patients and increases in the number of male patients, especially white men over the age of forty-five.[159] Not until 1955 did patient numbers at Waverly Hills start to steadily decrease due to combinations of multidrug therapy, surgical procedures, and outpatient treatment. Throughout the 1940s and 1950s, Waverly Hills administrators expanded patient services and programs, with the aim of helping patients to learn new skills, cope with family and personal problems, and endure their time at the sanatorium until they were discharged.

PATIENT ADMISSIONS AND DEPARTURES IN THE 1940s

After taking over management of Waverly Hills Sanatorium in 1942, the Board of Health began to limit the types of patients admitted to the institution. Administrators and medical staff curtailed the admission of school-aged children, due to studies showing that children with incipient cases were not likely to be infectious and could be cared for just as well in their homes as in the sanatorium. The number of children at the sanatorium declined sharply, with only one child admitted in 1947. In 1948, the administration announced

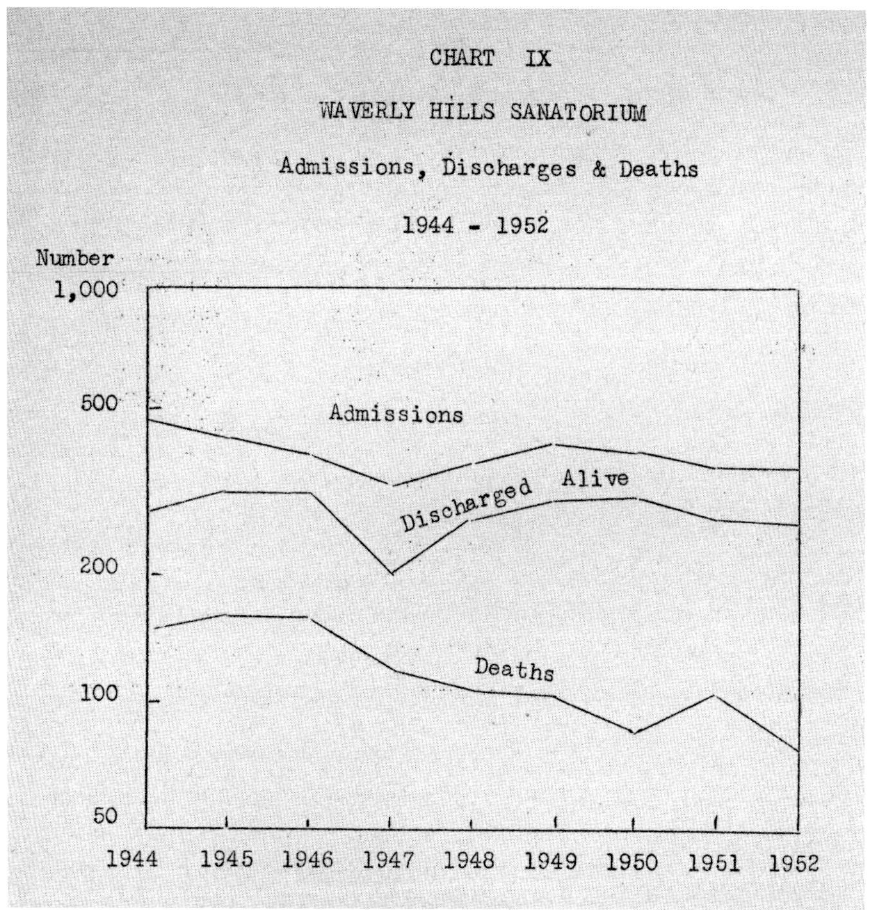

A chart showing a post–World War II dip and then a leveling out of admissions to Waverly Hills Sanatorium through 1952, with an overall decline in the number of deaths. *Louisville–Jefferson County Board of Health, 1952 annual report, Kornhauser Health Sciences Library, University of Louisville.*

it was limiting the admission of "observation cases, non-tuberculous cases" and "strictly custodial cases" among adult patients, indicating that such cases previously had been admitted to the sanatorium.[160]

As the Waverly Hills administration and medical staff restricted who was admitted to the sanatorium, they were also dealing with the ongoing problem of patients who left the sanatorium without the approval of physicians. The institution often had a waiting list, but it also always had patients who checked themselves out before their course of treatment was completed or before they died. A study of patients who left Waverly Hills against physicians' advice in 1942 attributed departures in part to high turnover in the medical staff during World War II. Other reasons, such as homesickness, economic difficulties, and childcare problems, were not unique to wartime conditions. The author of the study was Frances Fanelli, a University of Louisville graduate student. Fanelli was able to interview 43 of the 183 patients (or their family members) who left against their physicians' advice in 1942. Of these, 35 were white patients and 8 were Black patients, with more females than males overall.[161]

Fanelli's study provides a record of individuals struggling to balance the demands of institutional treatment with their desire to take care of their families or their own needs. "Mr. D.," the forty-four-year-old father of seven children, said he left the sanatorium because he was needed at home, where he could supervise the children while his wife worked. One of his children had been a "school delinquent" until he returned home. "Mrs. G.," whose case had been diagnosed as "minimal" right before she left Waverly Hills, told Fanelli her husband and children had been managing well without her, but she thought her husband was giving the children too many responsibilities. "Mr. E." found out while he was at Waverly Hills that his wife had been unfaithful to him. He left Waverly Hills to try to work on their relationship, but she insisted on a divorce. He remained away from the sanatorium to finalize the divorce and arrangements for their children.[162]

The wife of "Mr. W.," who had deserted his family after deserting Waverly Hills Sanatorium, said her husband had not improved during his hospitalization. The "quiet routine" of the sanatorium had been too slow for her husband, who before his time at Waverly Hills had led a busy life as a restaurant owner and gambler. Another patient, "Mrs. F," a sixty-seven-year-old woman, also could not endure institutional life. Her home life had not been lively—she lived "a lonely life" with another older woman, punctuated with infrequent visits from her son, grandson, and nephew. But she thought her occasional interaction with her housemate and her family was better than her even more isolated life at Waverly Hills.[163]

Some patients left because they did not feel sick or have serious symptoms or because they preferred to seek treatment outside the sanatorium. Significantly, thirty of the forty-three patients in Fanelli's study continued to receive medical attention after they left the sanatorium. Most obtained treatment or nursing services from the Waverly Hills Tuberculosis Clinic, but ten of them—all white patients—put themselves under the care of private physicians. "Mr. H." remained at Waverly Hills for five months before he left against the advice of his physicians. He said his chart had listed his diagnosis as "moderately-advanced tuberculosis," but his sputum tests were negative and his condition was listed as "active improved." He sought treatment from a private physician after leaving. "Mr. C." objected to an operation recommended to him, and he thought he had received "poor treatment" at the sanatorium. After leaving, he underwent the operation at the hands of a physician whom he trusted and "his condition improved."[164]

In April 1945, Waverly Hills obtained its first full-time social worker, one of the recommendations made in Fanelli's study. The social worker tried to help patients manage their financial and family issues back home while they remained at Waverly Hills. Among the first patients attended to by the social worker were a thirty-five-year-old woman who had three young children at home and a woman whose husband said she was not really sick and demanded that she leave the sanatorium.[165]

SANATORIUM ACTIVITIES AND FAMILY VISITS

Boosting morale among patients who spent months and years at the sanatorium had been a key part of the therapeutic regimen at Waverly Hills since its founding. The recreational, educational, and occupational services offered at Waverly Hills were seen as critical to helping patients recover their health and transition back to life outside the sanatorium. According to the Board of Health, "These are activities which stimulate patients to want to get well."[166] Waverly Hills administrators ramped up these programs in the postwar period and addressed some of the vast racial disparities that had always existed between the amenities provided in the main sanatorium for white patients and those in the hospital for Black patients. What remained restricted for all patients after World War II were forbidden items like alcohol, the times and days family and friends could visit them, and the passes giving them official leave from the sanatorium.

In the postwar years, Waverly Hills officials expanded services for Black patients while continuing to maintain racially segregated facilities. During World War II, white patients in the main sanatorium had a full-time librarian who ran the library and visited bed-bound patients to let them choose from her cart of books. Meanwhile, patients in the Black hospital organized their own "Waverly's Readers Club" in which members paid dues and ordered five magazines and a book each month. After finishing the reading materials, the club donated them to the Black hospital's small library. In 1946, the Board of Health arranged with the Louisville Free Public Library to help the

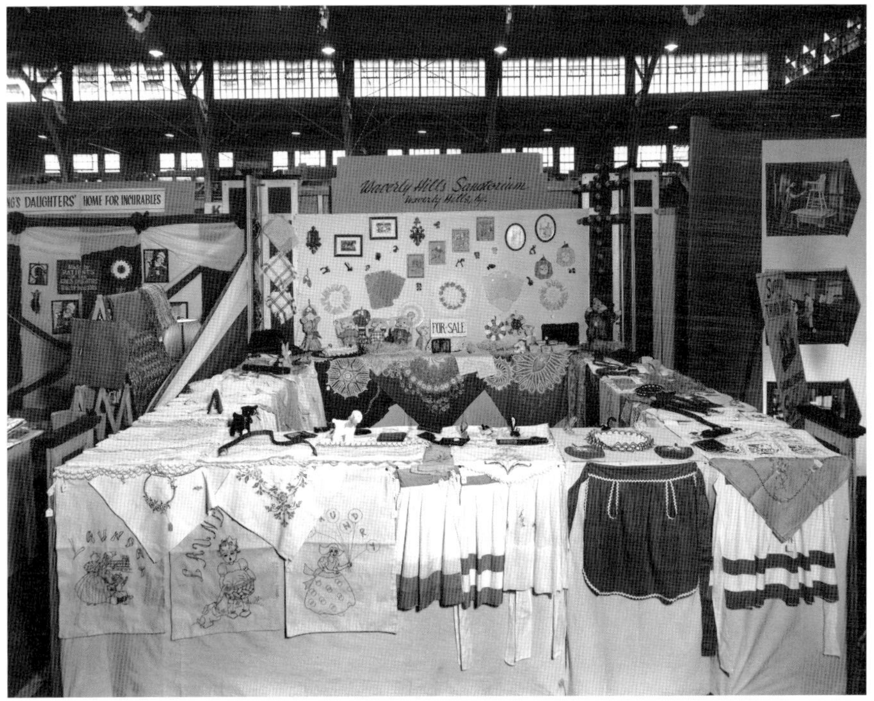

Waverly Hills Sanatorium exhibit of occupational therapy goods at the Kentucky state fair, 1950. *ULPA CS 255406, Archives and Special Collections, University of Louisville.*

Waverly Hills library department increase its offering of reading material to patients, "especially in the colored unit."[167]

The Board of Health's 1946 annual report was the first to provide statistics on the number of Black patients served by the Waverly Hills occupational therapy program, which offered instruction and classes to patients who were limited to their beds as well as to patients who could do work in the occupational therapy shop. In 1946, the program was staffed with "two occupational therapists in the white unit and one in the colored unit." The total number of patients served was 417, with 216 white bed patients, 65 white shop patients, 100 Black bed patients and 36 Black shop patients.[168]

Connected with the occupational therapy program at Waverly Hills were rehabilitation services. In 1938, the Louisville Tuberculosis Association established a rehabilitation program in the city to help patients discharged from the sanatorium find jobs appropriate for their physical condition. Beginning in 1944, the association's rehabilitation counselor, Catherine B. Richardson, began to make regular visits to Waverly Hills, and she soon worked with both white and Black patients.[169] Rosetta Squires had been a patient at the Black hospital for two and a half years in the mid-1940s. With the assistance of Richardson and with classes offered through the Louisville Board of Education, Squires received her high school diploma. When she expressed interest in nursing, Richardson helped her start a position as a part-time practical nurse at Waverly Hills after she was discharged as a patient. Later in the 1950s, she attended the Louisville General Hospital nursing school.[170] Richardson also helped Carl Liggin enter the ministry of the African Methodist Episcopal Church after his first hospitalization at Waverly Hills, and the Louisville Tuberculosis Association contributed to his tuition at Ohio's Payne Theological Seminary. In 1953, Liggin had to leave the seminary to return for a second hospitalization at Waverly Hills, and he was currently taking typing classes so he could prepare inspirational material for fellow patients.[171]

Female patients and some male patients in the main sanatorium were offered home economics classes, as well as other educational and occupational therapy services. In 1953, Martha Thomas wrote about Waverly Hills as a "haven of rest" during her thirteen months there, and she expressed gratitude for the rehabilitation program that prepared her for "home life again."[172] In 1957, the rehabilitation program turned an unfinished storeroom in the main sanatorium into a "model apartment," complete with living, dining, and laundry rooms, and "an almost-automatic kitchen" with all the latest equipment. The program was funded by the Kentucky State Bureau of Rehabilitation Services, the Louisville Tuberculosis Association, and a federal grant from the Department of Health, Education, and Welfare. Students included not just women but also "men who plan to help their working wives with the housework." Four of the male students had just learned to whip up cupcakes with coconut frosting.[173]

Visiting times and holiday passes gave patients the chance to connect with family and friends outside the sanatorium, but these opportunities were limited. Many patients and family members said their time apart from each other was the worst part of sanatorium treatment, though some patients may have appreciated a break from home or work life. In 1945, patients who were physically well enough to leave the sanatorium were offered forty-eight-hour passes four times a year—at Thanksgiving, Christmas, Easter, and Fourth of July.[174] When Jeri Gordon Brown talked with Louisville historian Tom Owen about the three and a half years her mother spent at the Black hospital at Waverly Hills in the 1940s, she remembered as significant the point at which her mother finally received passes to go home and see her children.[175]

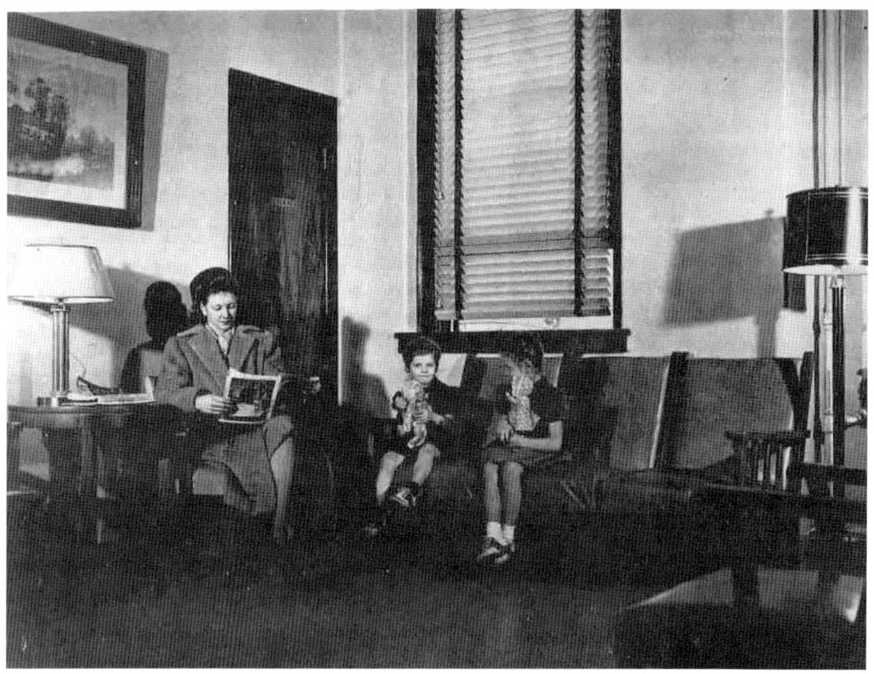

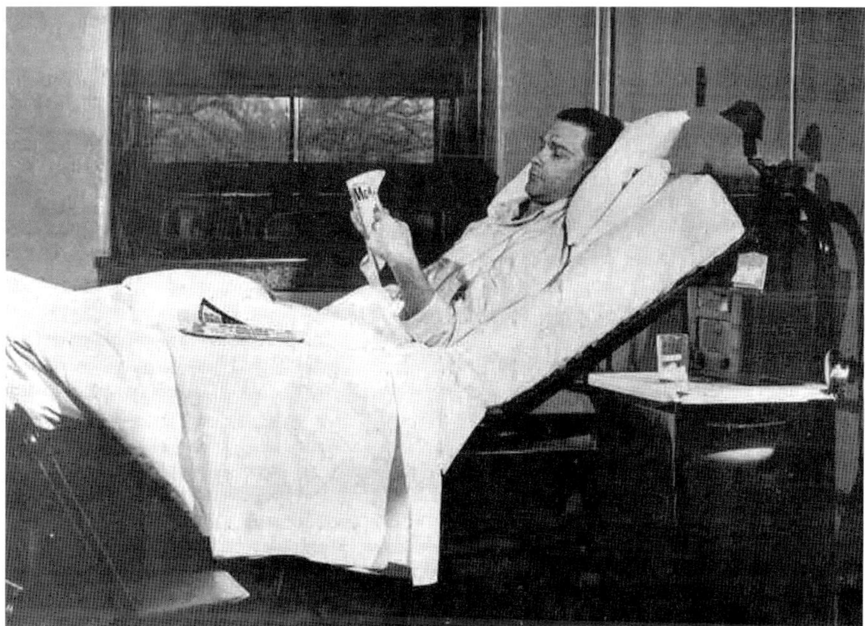

This page: The visitors' waiting room and patient room in the main sanatorium. *Louisville–Jefferson County Board of Health, 1947 annual report, Kornhauser Health Sciences Library, University of Louisville.*

In the 1940s, family members or friends of patients could go to Waverly Hills during twice-a-week visiting hours. When Pauline King's husband was at Waverly Hills in 1944, she made the "long trek" from eastern Jefferson County with their one-year-old child to visit him every Sunday and on holidays, making multiple bus transfers for every trip. Along the way, she made friends with other young women traveling to see their loved ones at the sanatorium.[176] Carol Miller Goodlett was eight years old when her mother entered Waverly Hills, and she remembered her family's visits ending in distress for her mother: "She would be so upset after we would leave that the doctor suggested only a visitation of once a month." In 1948, her mother died at the main sanatorium at the age of twenty-nine.[177]

Some patients were allowed more visitors or amenities due to a special occasion or their social stature. For the seventeenth birthday of Waverly Hills patient Charles Hardy in 1955, he was visited by fifty members of the teenage choir from his church, Victory Memorial Baptist. His mother and stepfather brought him a birthday cake, a fried chicken dinner, and a dozen records for him to play on his phonograph in his room. His friends took up a collection to buy him a television set.[178] In the early 1950s, nineteen-year-old Larry Weatherby—son of Kentucky governor Lawrence W. Weatherby—was given a private room on the wing of the first floor of the main sanatorium. Waverly Hills physician Dr. J. Frank W. Stewart said Larry had a "not so serious case" of tuberculosis and received a private room for security reasons for his parents' visits. The nurses alerted Dr. Stewart about some of the patients on Larry's wing drinking and "having too much fun" during the evenings. Larry had a small refrigerator in the corner of his room, which he told Dr. Stewart was for soft drinks and "special foods his mom would bring him." After Dr. Stewart checked and found cans of beer, he took away the refrigerator. Dr. Stewart noted that rather than holding a grudge against him (and possibly wanting to avoid any publicity getting out about the fridge stocked with beer), Larry gave him a leather jewelry box upon his discharge from the sanatorium, and his parents invited Dr. Stewart and his wife to Larry's wedding a few years later.[179]

ANTIBIOTICS, MULTIDRUG THERAPY, AND SURGERY

Speaking at a medical meeting in 1946, Dr. John J. Phair, director of the local health department, emphasized the need for more aggressive preventative measures and treatments for tuberculosis. The costs of hospitalization continued to rise, he pointed out, and there was a shift in

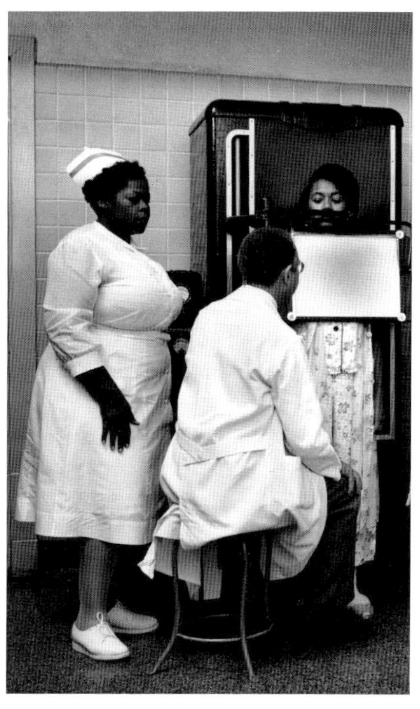

Nurse Alma Stamps and Dr. Orville Ballard examining a patient with a fluoroscope, December 1955. *Courtesy of* Louisville Courier-Journal.

medical thinking away from "merely keeping a patient flat on his back indefinitely and hoping he'll get well." He said the newly developed Bacillus Calmette-Guerin (BCG) vaccine would help prevent tuberculosis, and various surgical procedures would help discharge patients more quickly from sanatoriums. Ultimately, the BCG vaccine was not widely used in the United States due to questions about its efficacy, and public health officials relied more on case finding and contact tracing to try to prevent the spread of tuberculosis. For the treatment of tuberculosis, physicians would turn to a combination of surgery and new antibiotics and drugs.[180]

Streptomycin, discovered in 1943, was the first antibiotic found to be effective in treating certain forms of tuberculosis, but it took a decade of physicians combining antibiotics with other drugs before patients experienced consistently favorable results. In Louisville and Jefferson County, the Board of Health first reported on streptomycin's promise in 1946. According to Dr. Morris Weiss Jr., Dr. Jesse Bell was one of the first to be given streptomycin at Waverly Hills. Dr. Bell had been diagnosed with tuberculosis and, until 1947, worked on the medical staff of the Black hospital at Waverly Hills, in addition to his responsibilities as director at the Central Louisville Health Center.[181]

In 1948, the *Courier-Journal* reported results of the use of streptomycin at Waverly Hills as "gratifying" but also "disappointing" in many cases. Many patients developed resistance to streptomycin and at times negatively reacted to its toxicity. "Streptomycin is no cure-all," cautioned the article, but rather an additional weapon in the fight against tuberculosis.[182] In the early 1950s, physicians began to report success treating patients suffering from advanced tuberculosis with a multidrug combination of isonicotinic-acid compounds (also known as isoniazid or INH) with streptomycin or para-aminosalicylic acid (PAS).[183]

X-RAY REPORT

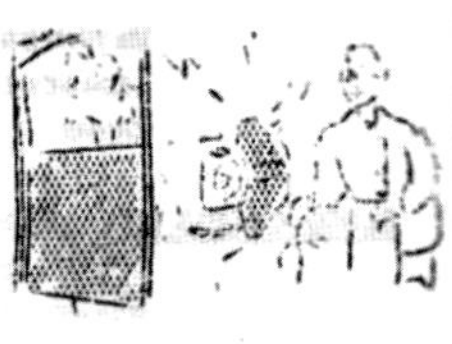

THE X-RAY REPORT GIVEN ON THE FOLLOWING PAGE DIFFERS FROM PREVIOUS REPORTS IN THAT "NUMBER OF PATIENTS" IS LISTED RATHER THAN "NUMBER OF FILMS USED." THEREFORE, NO COMPARATIVE FIGURES WILL BE GIVEN. WAVERLY HILLS SANATORIUM IS FORTUNATE IN HAVING COMPLETE X-RAY EQUIPMENT, INCLUDING EQUIPMENT FOR MAKING PLANIGRAMS.

THE NEW ELECTROCARDIOGRAPHIC UNIT AND BASAL METABOLISM UNIT HAVE BEEN SET UP IN THE X-RAY DEPARTMENT FOR CONVENIENCE. THE X-RAY TECHNICIANS WILL BE INSTRUCTED IN THE USE OF THE ELECTROCARDIOGRAPHIC UNIT. ARRANGEMENTS FOR INTERPRETATION BY COMPETENT CARDIOLOGISTS HAVE BEEN MADE.

NUMBER CHEST X-RAYS, SANATORIUM PATIENTS		2299
NUMBER CHEST X-RAYS, SANATORIUM EMPLOYEES		257
NUMBER CHEST X-RAYS, OUT-PATIENTS (PNEUMO.)		230
NUMBER PLANIGRAMS, SANATORIUM PATIENTS		200
NUMBER BRONCHOGRAMS		33
NUMBER PYELOGRAMS		16
NUMBER GASTRO-INTESTINAL EXAMINATIONS		87
NUMBER BARIUM ENEMAS		29
NUMBER DENTAL PATIENTS		74
MISCELLANEOUS X-RAYS, SANATORIUM PATIENTS		122
MISCELLANEOUS X-RAYS, SANATORIUM EMPLOYEES		39
LIPIODOL INJECTIONS (SINUS CASES)		15
TOTAL X-RAYS TAKEN		3401
FLUOROSCOPIC EXAMINATIONS OF CHEST		11005
PATIENTS IN SANATORIUM	8177	
OUT-PATIENT PNEUMO CASES	2828	
GASTRO-INTESTINAL FLUOROSCOPIC EXAMINATIONS		328

X-ray report for Waverly Hills Sanatorium, 1946. *Louisville–Jefferson County Board of Health, 1946 annual report, Kornhauser Health Sciences Library, University of Louisville.*

The number of surgical procedures at Waverly Hills increased during the same years physicians were trying streptomycin and other drugs on patients. In 1946, Waverly Hills medical staff reported that "collapse therapy, especially that of artificial pneumothorax, continues to be our most productive form of treatment." A select number of patients underwent more invasive surgical procedures such as thoracoplasty (removing some of the patient's ribs to collapse the diseased cavities of a patient's lung) and the "more radical" lobectomy or pneumonectomy (removing diseased parts of a lung or an entire lung). In the late 1940s, physicians reported that streptomycin helped some patients in the advanced stages of tuberculosis to improve enough to undergo those procedures.[184]

The surgical program at Waverly Hills expanded in the postwar years, but it also faced problems of space and staffing. In 1949, the operating room was outfitted with air conditioning and space was made for a new air-conditioned autopsy room. In 1953, the surgery department took over the solarium on the fourth floor to use as a surgical ward. Due to staffing struggles, the Board of Health contracted with the University of Louisville School of Medicine for a surgeon and surgical resident to do operations at Waverly Hills.[185]

By the mid-1950s, Waverly Hills was touting the success of a program of multidrug therapy and surgery. In the 1954–55 fiscal year, patients underwent a total of 323 surgical operations and were given 28,300 vials of streptomycin, 2,500,00 tablets of PAS, and 144,000 capsules of INH. Waverly Hills administrators and medical staff claimed these treatments helped shorten periods of hospitalization at the sanatorium:

> *It is not easy for any patient with tuberculosis to accept the long term bed rest most vital in the treatment of the disease because of the psychological problems, the separation from loved ones and the financial burdens which become particularly acute when the patient is the bread winner. With surgery and the new wonder drugs, the length of stay is shortened and some previously hopeless cases can be cured.*[186]

In February 1956, the sanatorium was able to discharge thirty longtime patients. They were tasked with continuing their drug therapy at home and returning every month to the sanatorium to see a physician and every three months to have a chest X-ray made. In October, the Board of Health

SURGICAL REPORT

THIS REPORT IS GIVEN FOR THE YEAR 1946, AND ON A COMPARATIVE BASIS FOR THE PREVIOUS FOUR YEARS.

REPORT FOR 1946

	PATIENTS	OPERATIONS
PNEUMONECTOMY	2	2
LOBECTOMY	2	2
EXTRAPLEURAL PNEUMOTHORAX	4	4
INTRAPLEURAL PNEUMONOLYSIS (CLOSED)	49	49
OPEN DRAINAGE	2	2
PHRENICS	19	19
MISCELLANEOUS (CHEST)	10	10
MISCELLANEOUS	5	5
TRANSFUSIONS	56	103
THORACOPLASTY	43	74

FIRST STAGE – 29 FOURTH STAGE – 5
SECOND STAGE – 28 FIFTH STAGE – 1
THIRD STAGE – 11

Surgical report for Waverly Hills Sanatorium, 1946. *Louisville–Jefferson County Board of Health, 1946 annual report, Kornhauser Health Sciences Library, University of Louisville.*

established an outpatient treatment clinic at the Waverly Hills Clinic (which had moved to 240 East Madison Street earlier in the decade) for tuberculosis patients discharged from Waverly Hills Sanatorium or from the Veterans Administration Hospital.[187]

Two patients who received a combination of treatments at Waverly Hills in the early 1950s and made it out of the sanatorium to live long lives were Margaret Baugh and Evelyn Knight Helm. Margaret Baugh had her story of her time at Waverly Hills recorded by Steve Russell Video Productions in 2017, when she was ninety-one years old. Born in 1926, Baugh was a young woman in her mid-twenties when she received an X-ray at the telephone company where she worked. When the X-ray showed indications of pulmonary tuberculosis, she was told to go to Waverly Hills, where she remained from April 1950 through September 1951. She was treated by Dr. Elmars Spunde, whom she said "was a really good doctor." But she dreaded the pneumothorax treatments that she underwent on a regular basis for over six months. They were uncomfortable and made her feel like she was going to smother. According to someone who knew her later in life and who commented on the video interview, she had also undergone surgery to remove a diseased part of her lung while at Waverly Hills.[188]

For Margaret Baugh, the most heartbreaking part of her hospitalization was having to leave her young son Mike. Physicians initially said she would only need to remain at the sanatorium for a few months, but she ended up staying there a year and a half. She said her emotional state when she was told she needed to stay longer was "really low" and nearly unbearable. Her husband moved to Logan County and visited less often, and it was hard for her to only be able to visit her family four times a year with the holiday passes. The sanatorium food was "reasonably good" except for the bread, and her husband would bring her hot dogs and raisin bread that she cooked with her toaster in her room "until it smelled up the whole floor." She read books from the main sanatorium's "wonderful library" and learned to crochet in the occupational therapy shop. She said patients were rolled out of their rooms in May onto the sun porch and were not brought in until it snowed later in the year. She enjoyed looking out the screened windows of the sun porch, but the cold was miserable even with layers of clothing and blankets. Over the course of her time at Waverly Hills, she was able to increase her weight from about 110 to more than 180 pounds. When she left Waverly Hills in the early fall of 1951, she felt like she had been let out of jail.

Evelyn Knight Helm's time at Waverly Hills partially overlapped with the months Margaret Baugh was there. Helm was the oldest daughter of a

In this grate land of ours there
a place call Waverly Hills.
It was on Oct 2. 1950, time 3 P.M
The whistle blew, the Chatter begin
A New Girl just Came in, Room No 244
Now on this day May 29, 1951,
there has been More Chatter, the
Girl in 244, dont Know North
South East or West.
To get attention she see's
Tray Bay's in the tree tops.
When on the Farm and
here a Little face Think of Me
Billie Richmond

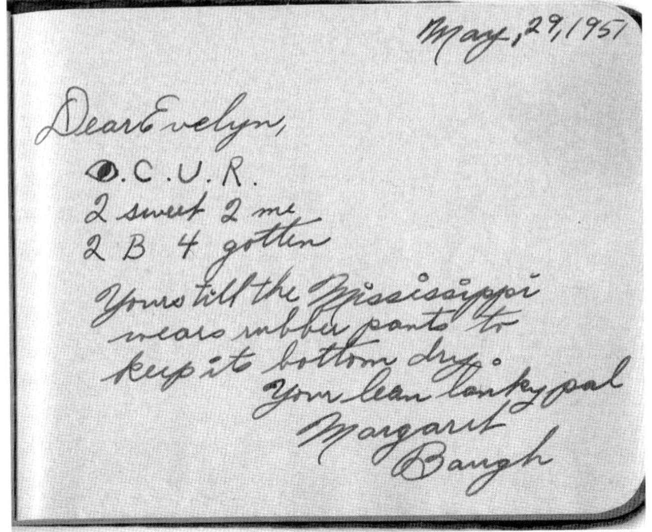

May, 29, 1951

Dear Evelyn,
I.C.U.R.
2 sweet 2 me
2 B 4 gotten
Yours till the Mississippi
wears rubber pants to
keep its bottom dry.
Your lean lanky pal
Margaret Baugh

This page: Evelyn Knight Helm autograph book, May 29, 1951 entries. *Mss. C H, Filson Historical Society.*

farmer and his wife from eastern Kentucky. Like Baugh, Helm's story began with a diagnosis at her workplace. In 1950, she was twenty years old and working at Louisville's American Tobacco Company, which manufactured Lucky Strike cigarettes. When one of her coworkers was diagnosed with tuberculosis, the rest of the employees were screened for the disease, and Helm tested positive. She was admitted to Waverly Hills Sanatorium in October. Like Baugh, Helm also had Dr. Elmars Spunde as her physician. In early January 1951, Dr. Spunde and another physician removed the diseased lower lobe of Helm's lung. She remained at the sanatorium until she was discharged in November, a few months after Baugh.[189]

One of the items carried out of Waverly Hills by Evelyn Knight Helm was a small leather-bound autograph book. On its pages are personal notes and inspirational sayings for Helm from other patients, female and male. The messages bear witness to the many people Helm met before she was discharged and able to make "the walk down the hill." Billie Richmond wrote in the autograph book in May 1951, recalling the first day Helm arrived at the sanatorium: "It was on Oct. 2 1950, time 3 PM. The whistle blew. The chatter began. A new girl just came in, Room No. 244." Dorothy Chapman wrote a teasing note to Helm: "If you dream of heaven and all its joys, Think more of the Bible and less of the boys." On November 17, Dorothy Hudson bid her friend goodbye: "Dear Evelyn, Sure has been nice walking the hill with you. Here's hoping we both make the grade next Wednesday!"[190]

One entry in Helm's autograph book was written on May 29, 1951, and signed, "Your lean lanky pal Margaret Baugh." Out of the hundreds of white patients in the main sanatorium—an average of 265 patients a day in 1950–51—Helm and Baugh met each other and crossed paths enough times to lead to Baugh writing a charming note in Helm's book. Among Margaret Baugh's many recollections of the emotional and physical distress she experienced during her months at Waverly Hills was a positive memory, one about the "wonderful friends" she made at the sanatorium, three of whom she was especially close to, and one of them a Catholic like herself. We do not know if Helm was one of Baugh's fondly recollected friends, but it is clear that such relationships helped patients to endure the long months of institutional treatment.

Chapter 8

THE LAST YEARS OF WAVERLY HILLS SANATORIUM

Beginning in the mid-1940s, Louisville and Jefferson County health officials began to press the Kentucky State Tuberculosis Hospital Commission to provide financial support for or take over the management of Waverly Hills Sanatorium. The commission oversaw six tuberculosis districts throughout Kentucky, each served by one of six state-funded and state-run sanatoriums: Hazelwood Sanatorium in Louisville and five new sanatoriums built between 1946 and 1950 in Madisonville, Paris, Ashland, London, and Glasgow. In 1952, after the local Board of Health warned that Waverly Hills might need to close due to budget problems, the state made its first appropriation, providing $200,000 a year while the city and county contributed a total of approximately $500,000 a year. As the State Tuberculosis Hospital Commission put off deciding whether to take over Waverly Hills Sanatorium, the Board of Health continued to manage the institution through the 1950s.[191]

RECALCITRANT PATIENTS AND FINAL DEBATES

One major issue in the 1950s shaping debates over the future of Waverly Hills Sanatorium was the problem of "recalcitrant patients"—patients with active cases of tuberculosis who refused to undergo or remain in treatment. For decades, health officials had pushed for the legal ability to forcibly hospitalize such patients. In 1954, Kentucky passed a law outlining penalties of up to a $500 fine and a six-month jail sentence for people with active cases of tuberculosis who refused to cooperate with institutional treatment and who were deemed a public hazard. If they agreed to be admitted for sanatorium treatment, their fine and jail sentence were suspended.[192]

The law was tested for the first time in Louisville in May 1955. In the Bowman Field housing project, neighbors alerted welfare workers about navy veteran Hugh Swift. Swift was the thirty-three-year-old father of seven young children, and like many veterans, he had contracted tuberculosis during his military service in either World War II or the Korean War. Saying he was worried about his family, Swift had repeatedly left the Veterans Administration tuberculosis hospital in Outwood, Kentucky, against medical advice. After three of his children tested positive for tuberculosis, a warrant was filed for his arrest. The county court found Swift guilty of violating the 1954 state law and ordered him to six months of treatment at Waverly Hills Sanatorium.[193]

Health officials quickly discovered that the state law to punish or hospitalize recalcitrant patients was almost impossible to enforce. Jails had no facilities for treating tuberculosis, so the imprisonment of a tuberculosis patient posed a threat to the health of jail inmates and employees. The patient could be ordered to be admitted for sanatorium treatment, as Hugh Swift was, but in 1955, there was no locked ward to keep patients against their will at any tuberculosis sanatorium in the state.[194]

Waverly Hills administrators and staff lobbied for the establishment of a locked ward as well as for programs to help keep patients in the sanatorium. In 1958, Waverly Hills medical director Dr. Alvin Mullen requested funding for a security ward from the Board of Health, saying that 25 to 40 percent of patients left the sanatorium against medical advice. He claimed these patients were the main reason for the continuing high case rates of tuberculosis in Kentucky in comparison with the rest of the country. Waverly Hills social worker Ruth Edwards recommended the implementation of an Alcoholics Anonymous program and psychiatric treatment at the sanatorium, citing a three-year study she had conducted showing that most recalcitrant patients were white men who left due to their struggles with alcoholism, family and financial problems, or a "refusal to admit they were sick."[195]

Waverly Hills never got its locked ward, but the state-run Hazelwood Sanatorium did in 1959. Hazelwood, located on Bluegrass Avenue in Louisville and managed by the State Tuberculosis Hospital Commission, served a tuberculosis district consisting of twenty-six counties and performed all surgery for the state-run tuberculosis hospitals in Kentucky. Its locked ward was not entirely a success. Patients escaped, with some slipping down drainpipes, one locking up a nurse in the toilet closet and running off, and another taking the bus back to his hometown of Harlan still in his pajamas. The state planned to hire guards around the clock and to put bars on the windows of the units.[196]

Late in the summer of 1959, the State Tuberculosis Hospital Commission signaled its willingness to take over the care of patients at Waverly Hills. A public debate erupted over whether Waverly Hills or Hazelwood should be closed if their patient populations were combined. In July, Waverly Hills had 280 of its 400 beds filled with patients, and Hazelwood had 180 of its 307 beds filled. Many people pushed for Waverly Hills to remain open, saying more resources, not less, were needed in the continuing fight against tuberculosis. In October, superintendent S.A. Ruskjer said 56.5 percent of patients admitted at Waverly Hills in the past year had a diagnosis of far-advanced tuberculosis, showing that the disease was still serious. In early 1960, Ruskjer told the Board of Health that all of the beds at the sanatorium would be put to use if they could get "the patients who have left the Sanatorium against medical advice to return."[197]

The State Tuberculosis Hospital Commission and other state officials made clear their preference for transferring Waverly Hills patients to Hazelwood Sanatorium. They said Hazelwood, not Waverly Hills, had a security ward, and recalcitrant patients who refused treatment would always be a problem and push up rates of the disease. Thomas Layton, the executive director of the State Tuberculosis Hospital Commission, said "money could be better spent on rehabilitation, social work, education, and occupational activities for the patients who will accept hospitalization" than on keeping open two sanatoriums in Louisville with many beds remaining empty. He and other officials preferred Hazelwood's location in the city, which was more accessible to employees.[198]

In January 1960, Kentucky governor Bert Combs issued an official recommendation to the state legislature to close Waverly Hills Sanatorium and transfer patients to Hazelwood.[199] Governor Combs's announcement set off a slew of letters to the *Courier-Journal* from former patients and employees making their case to save Waverly Hills. Many saw Waverly Hills as a better institution than Hazelwood for the care of patients. It had private and semi-private rooms, whereas Hazelwood had mostly wards. M.T. Jones said Hazelwood barely had walking space between its beds: "There is no comfort sitting in bed, certainly not eating in it, no exercises, no way to breathe deeply, to expand and develop the lower part of their lungs." Others credited Waverly Hills with saving their lives and praised the institution's "excellent care," "trained personnel in therapy and rehabilitation," and "restful atmosphere of efficiency and beauty." Anna Laird recalled of her two hospitalizations at the sanatorium, "When you go to Waverly Hills your heartaches are their heartaches also."[200] A graduate nurse who had worked at Waverly Hills provided a florid description of the institution's spirit-lifting surroundings:

> *There is a majesty, grandeur, and dignity in its high-upon-a-hill location. It gives one a feeling that all need to reach upward for the intangible things of the spirit. There is beauty everything the eyes roam. Blue birds singing outside your window, bring happiness and harmony so necessary in the recovery of the sick. There are life-giving trees that fill one with awe and wonder and create in our inmost selves a oneness with our Heavenly Father, "for only God can make a tree."*[201]

Others questioned the therapeutic value of Waverly Hill's open spaces. In 1955, an editorial in the *Courier-Journal* explained how surgery and multidrug therapy lessened the importance of fresh air in the treatment of tuberculosis: "Patients hospitalized in a new modern wing of General Hospital would do quite as well as they now do in the open spaces that surround Waverly, if not better."[202] In the fall of 1959, Jefferson County resident Earl J. Krebs wrote a letter to the *Courier-Journal* to question how fresh the air around Waverly Hills really was: "Now they have new drugs and surgery, but the nice, clean, fresh air is no more." Krebs noted how wind from the south carried smoke and dust from the Kosmosdale cement works. Wind from the west carried smoke from the Louisville Gas and Electric Company plant. Wind from the north carried ash, fumes, and gases from Rubbertown oil refineries. And wind from the east carried the smells of the Waverly Hills incinerator and the hog farm, "where they feed the garbage from Waverly and General Hospital to upwards of 300 heads of hog." Additional smoke came from Dixie Highway homes and businesses burning coal and oil in the winter months. Similar to Waverly Hills, Hazelwood Sanatorium used to be located in "nice, clean, open country" but now found itself in the middle of a congested suburb. Installing air conditioning in one of the tuberculosis institutions was one solution, Krebs suggested. Or the federal government could cooperate with the states to open a sanatorium for patients out west, "where it is known T.B. patients fare best."[203]

FAREWELL TO WAVERLY

In the spring of 1960, plans moved ahead for the expansion of Hazelwood and the closure of Waverly Hills. The renovation of Hazelwood, the transfer of Waverly Hills patients, the shutting down of the farm, and the letting go of employees would take well over a year. Deciding what to do with the sanatorium's aging facilities would take even longer. "Available soon: one hospital. Anybody want it?" asked a *Courier-Journal* article in reference to the main sanatorium.[204]

In 1960, Waverly Hills included twenty-two buildings on 544 acres, with 120 acres actively used for the sanatorium buildings and farm. The remaining acres were thickly wooded.[205] County officials and residents pressed for 300 acres of Waverly Hills to be given to the county parks and recreation department, asking pointedly, "Don't the people of Jefferson County own the land?" Board of Health member William Harrison, a

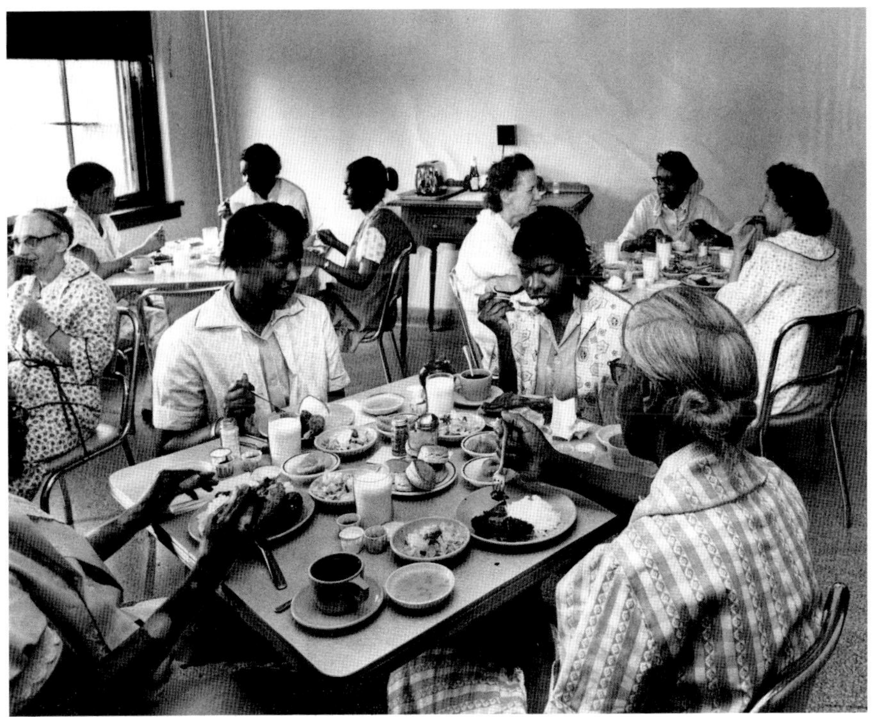

One of the small dining rooms in the main sanatorium of Waverly Hills, May 1960. A month later, the administration began to transfer patients to Hazelwood Sanatorium. *Courtesy of* Louisville Courier-Journal.

county resident, countered that city and not county funds had provided "the vast majority of the investment in Waverly Hills." The Board of Health expected more than $600,000 for the sale of Waverly Hills land abutting Dixie Highway for commercial development and along Pages Lane for residential development, and it was not going to give land away for free to the county. The county was able to secure funds from the Federal Housing Act of 1961 for the purchase of the land, and the 301-acre Waverly Hills Park opened in 1965.[206]

In June 1960, superintendent R.A. Ruskjer reported to the Board of Health that forty-four of the sixty patients "outside the main hospital" at Waverly Hills had been transferred to Hazelwood. The plan was for the rest of those sixty patients to be transferred by July 1, and all of the employees "serving the patient unit in process of transfer" would be laid off by July 15.[207] The board minutes did not specify what patient unit Ruskjer was referring to, but most certainly it was the hospital housing Black male patients and employing Black staff. One of the patients transferred to Hazelwood in this first shift was Andrew Jackson Spry, a Black patient who was either 105 or 106 years old. Spry had been admitted to Waverly Hills in September 1959 after a routine screening X-ray at General Hospital showed evidence of pulmonary tuberculosis. He reported getting along fine at Hazelwood, "now that he's convinced the cook is as good as the one he left behind" at Waverly Hills.[208]

The famed hog program at Waverly Hills came to a close in the fall of 1960, ending a long-standing arrangement in which the sanatorium collected not just General Hospital's garbage to feed the hogs but also General Hospital's "amputations." In September, S.A. Ruskjer informed General Hospital administrator John B. Buschemeyer that since the sanatorium was getting rid of its hogs, "we shall not be in position to use General Hospital's garbage after September 24, nor shall we be in position to haul amputations after that date."[209] He did not specify where the sanatorium had been hauling the amputated body parts.

By the end of October 1960, 82 employees from Waverly Hills had been laid off and the surgical program had been transferred to Hazelwood. The remaining 154 employees on the Waverly Hills staff outnumbered the 120 patients awaiting transfer while Hazelwood underwent renovation, but more employees were released in the months to come.[210]

With a bigger expansion underway at Hazelwood than originally intended, Waverly Hills continued to care for tuberculosis patients until the summer of 1961. Louisville architects Joseph and Joseph managed the Hazelwood

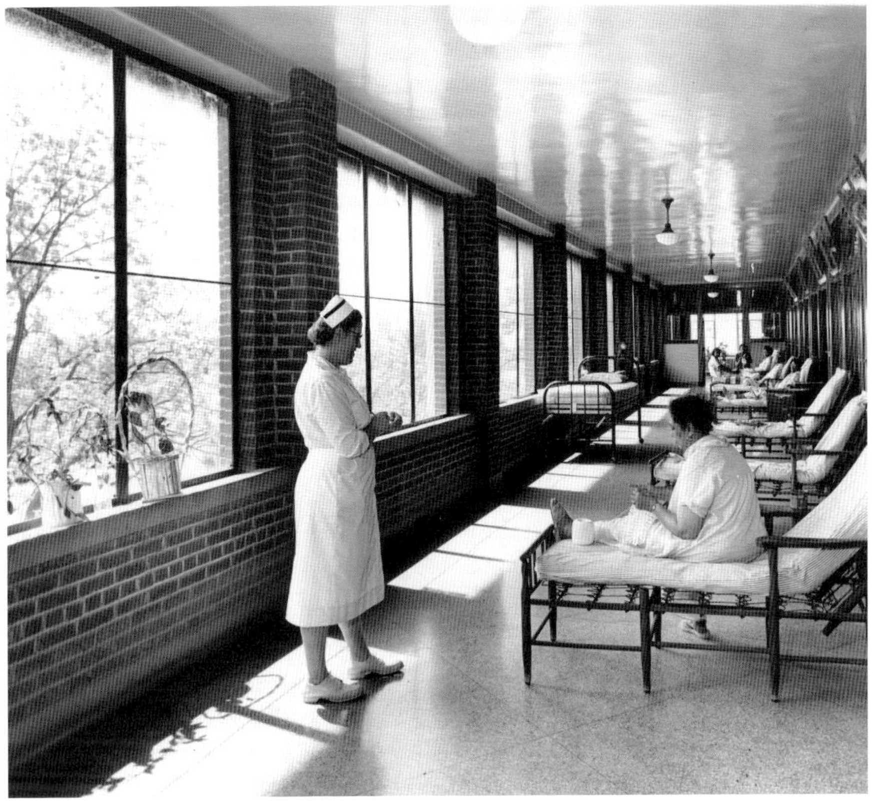

A nurse and a handful of patients on one of the main sanatorium's sun porches, May 1960. *Courtesy of* Louisville Courier-Journal.

renovation, with plans to convert wards into private and semiprivate patient rooms and to construct a three-story addition with "a home-economics training center, workshop, enlarged cafeteria, library, classrooms, and offices." The bed capacity was increased from 307 to 424. The renovation cost $920,000, with federal Hill-Burton hospital improvement funds contributing $139,778 of the total. Many people opposed to the closing of Waverly Hills questioned why so much money was spent to expand Hazelwood when Waverly Hills already had the facilities and beds being added to Hazelwood.[211]

The transfer of Waverly Hills patients to Hazelwood resumed in "small but frequent blocs" in March 1961. On June 2, a *Courier-Journal* editorial said the last patients had left Waverly Hills, "symbolizing an end and a beginning." The editorial credited taxpayers with contributing to a half-century-long battle against tuberculosis and praised Waverly Hills staff

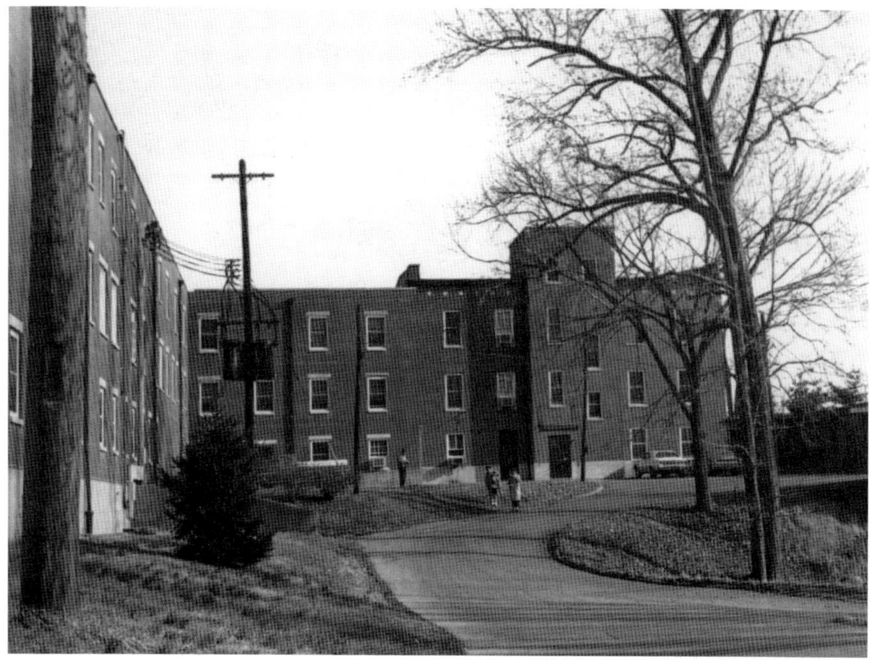

A rear view of Hazelwood Sanatorium in 1969, eight years after the completion of its renovation and addition. *HOS-51, Filson Historical Society.*

for its work over the years. It depicted the shift of patients to the state-run Hazelwood as a beneficial arrangement: "The patients are being transferred to a newer and more modern facility. The County is being relieved of a fixed expense."[212]

Dr. Orville Ballard and medical director Dr. Alvin Mullen had been at Waverly Hills since the 1920s and superintendent S.A. Ruskjer since the last year of World War II. Dr. Ballard joined the staff of the health department's tuberculosis clinic, and Dr. Mullen became director of tuberculosis control in the city and county. Ruskjer took on new professional positions but remained in his house on the grounds at Waverly Hills. In June 1961, he accepted a position as a consultant to the Kentucky State Tuberculosis Hospital Commission and to Seventh-day Adventist medical institutions in Michigan and Tennessee. In November, the seventy-two-year-old Ruskjer died of a heart attack at his Waverly Hills home.[213]

One of Ruskjer's last recommendations to the Board of Health in the summer of 1961 had been to hire security for Waverly Hills. He told the board, "As soon as it was known that Waverly Hills was going to be vacated, immediately attempted break ins, etc. had begun," with four teenagers

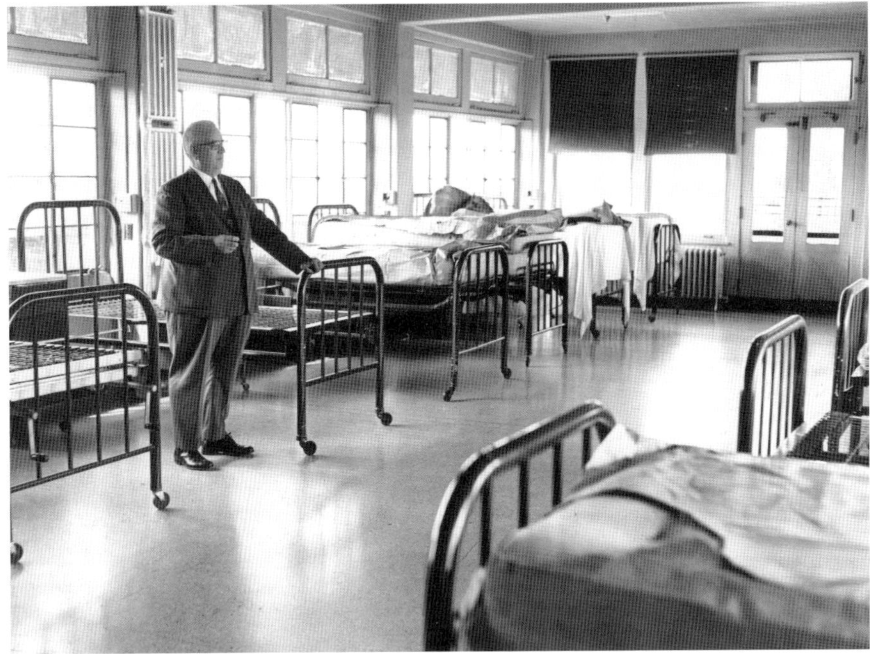

Dr. Alvin B. Mullen in a ward at Waverly Hills, with beds in the process of being stripped of their mattresses and sheets, May 1961. *Courtesy of* Louisville Courier-Journal.

arrested so far. The board contracted with a private company, Kentucky Security Police, hiring two men to work seven days a week for the following year. One covered the 3:00 to 11:00 p.m. shift, the other the 11:00 p.m. to 7:00 a.m. shift.[214]

In addition to these security officers patrolling the property, a small handful of employees continued to manage the grounds and facilities of Waverly Hills until the sanatorium complex was officially transferred to the Kentucky Department of Mental Health in July 1962. An administrative note preserved the names of the last Waverly Hills employees: Alva Arnold, Robert Noe, Goebel Miller, C. Clement Nevitt, William F. Paige, Rosco Allen, Charles K. Baker, and the farmers William Miller and Roy Thompson.[215] The release of the men from their jobs marked the end of Waverly Hills Sanatorium, which for over half a century had not just housed and treated tens of thousands of men, women, and children but also provided a place of work and residence to thousands of employees, many of them former patients.

In June 1962, a man who had been a patient at Waverly Hills twenty-five years earlier wrote to the *Courier-Journal* to say, "It was like losing a dear friend when reading about the closing." The writer remembered a series of roommates; some left apparently well, and others had "waited too long" to come to the sanatorium and "didn't make it." He concluded with a wistful goodbye to the sanatorium and lingering doubts about the decision to move patients to Hazelwood: "Farewell to Waverly, and good luck to the new hospital. I sincerely hope they know what they are doing."[216]

Chapter 9

DEATHS AND THE LEGACY OF WAVERLY HILLS SANATORIUM

In October 1962, over a year after the last patients had left Waverly Hills Sanatorium, the nonprofit Kentucky Geriatrics Foundation signed a lease with the state for the use of the main sanatorium building as a convalescent care facility for the aging. Originally called the Waverly Hills Geriatric Center, the facility was renamed Woodhaven Medical Services in 1970. After being investigated by the state for neglect of patients, Woodhaven closed in early 1981. Two years later, the property was listed in the National Register of Historic Places. Private investors during the next few decades pursued visions of turning the historic building into a prison or a paintball facility or erecting the world's tallest statue of Jesus on the grounds, but none of these ideas came to fruition. Teenagers and young adults claimed the abandoned building as a hangout as it fell into disrepair from vandalism and weather. Louisville resident Mark Johansen still bears a scar over the bridge of his nose from when he and his friends were exploring the old sanatorium in the early 1990s. After they heard police car sirens in the distance, Johansen scrambled to get out of the building through a broken window that left a cut on his face.[217]

Tina and Charles Mattingly bought the property in 2001 and undertook the colossal task of repairing and maintaining the last surviving building of Waverly Hills Sanatorium. The site is operated by the nonprofit Waverly Hills Historical Society and offers public tours and investigations. Popular interest in the building has grown in the past few decades, with television shows and internet sites fixating on paranormal activities and the infamous "death tunnel."[218]

The investigation of deaths at Waverly Hills Sanatorium—with the aim of understanding rather than sensationalizing its long history and mixed legacy—is an important endeavor. An examination of documented deaths and lives lost at Waverly Hills helps to illuminate past experiences and struggles at the institution's different buildings serving different groups of patients over the years.

One well-known fact about the broader history of Waverly Hills Sanatorium is that death rates from tuberculosis in the United States declined steadily throughout much of the twentieth century. In Louisville, the disease fell from the leading cause of death, with almost 250 deaths per 100,000 residents in 1910, to the twelfth-highest cause, with just under 15 deaths per 100,000 residents in 1959.[219] Tuberculosis was one of many infectious

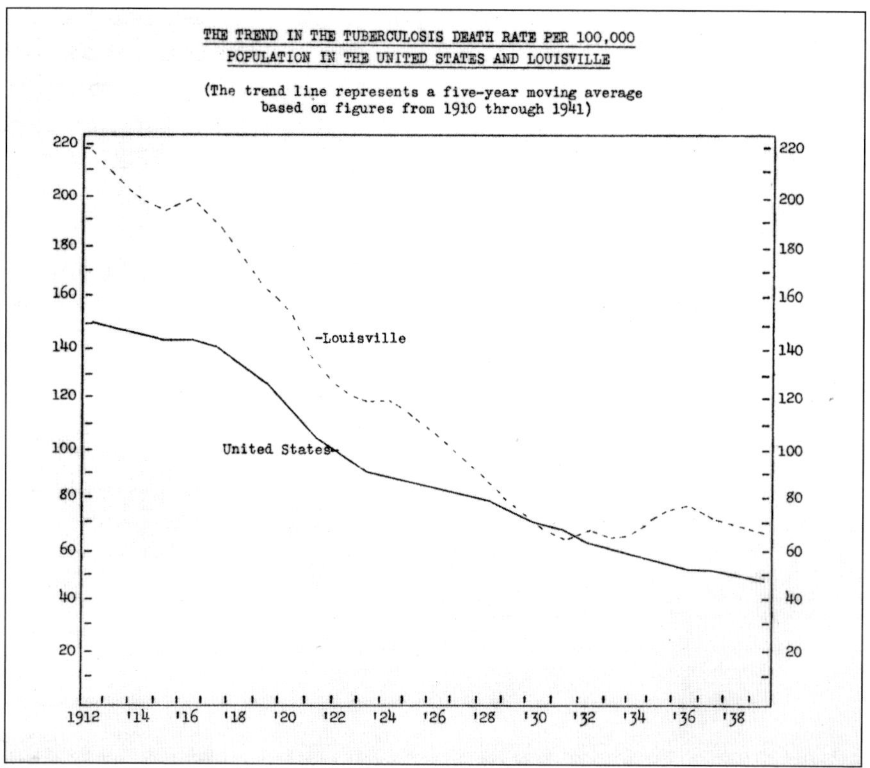

Above: Tuberculosis death rates declined through much of the twentieth century. *"Tuberculosis in Louisville," December 1942, Kornhauser Health Sciences Library, University of Louisville.*

Opposite: Louisville reported approximately 11,500 deaths from tuberculosis from 1907 to 1940. *Louisville Department of Health, 1940 annual report, Filson Historical Society.*

TUBERCULOSIS DEATHS BY NUMBER & RATES

LOUISVILLE (1907–1939)

YEAR	POPULATION	NO. OF DEATHS	RATES
1907	218,550	493	225.6
1908	220,450	479	217.3
1909	222,450	480	215.8
1910	223,928	542	242.0
1911	225,300	537	238.3
1912	226,450	479	211.5
1913	227,550	432	189.8
1914	228,700	499	218.2
1915	229,800	440	191.5
1916	230,050	435	189.0
1917	232,100	430	185.3
1918	233,200	509	218.3
1919	234,300	372	158.8
1920	238,450	333	139.7
1921	245,550	311	126.7
1922	252,700	328	129.8
1923	259,800	309	118.9
1924	266,900	297	111.3
1925	274,300	328	119.6
1926	281,150	335	119.3
1927	288,250	272	94.4
1928	295,350	227	76.9
1929	302,450	234	77.4
1930	307,745	224	72.8
1931	309,116	195	63.1
1932	310,213	172	55.4
1933	311,310	168	54.0
1934	312,407	279	89.3
1935	313,504	209	66.7
1936	314,601	233	74.1
1937	315,698	275	87.1
1938	316,795	237	74.8
1939	317,892	192	60.4
1940	318,989	191	59.8

diseases to undergo a decline in case and death rates beginning in the late nineteenth century. Decades before the introduction of antibiotics, a variety of factors including sanitation measures, increased natural resistance, and improved living standards helped reduce the spread of infectious diseases among many Americans.

It is difficult to measure the extent to which institutions like Waverly Hills Sanatorium contributed to this overall decline in tuberculosis rates.

Proponents of sanatorium treatment were targeting tuberculosis as a major source of death, and they understood how tuberculosis could be prevented. Public health advocates and officials were following sound medical principles at the time, aiming to isolate tuberculosis patients from the general public, provide education about disease transmission and hygienic practices, and build up the ability of patients to overcome the disease. Before the introduction of antibiotics and multidrug therapy in the 1940s and 1950s, there was no cure for tuberculosis, particularly for patients with advanced cases. A variety of lung collapse procedures, often called "barbaric" today, were among the only treatments enabling physicians to try to temporarily halt the progression of the disease in the lungs of patients, with the aim of increasing their chances of recovery.[220]

The number of deaths at Waverly Hills was distressingly high in many years—though nowhere close to the oft-cited and wildly inaccurate estimates of "a patient dying every hour" in the early years of Waverly Hills or of fifty thousand to sixty-four thousand deaths over the entire history of the institution.[221] Surviving statistics do not present a complete record of deaths at Waverly Hills, but reported numbers for different sets of years help to track trends and changes over time.

Statistics from the first five and a half years of Waverly Hills show that about a third of patients admitted also died there—almost certainly the highest proportion of deaths per total number of patients in the institution's history. The majority of admissions and deaths in these years were patients with advanced cases of tuberculosis who were housed first in tents in 1911–12 and then at the hospital that opened in January 1913 at Waverly Hills. A 1916 report identified 1,008 patients admitted to Waverly Hills from July 1910 to September 1914, 635 of whom were admitted as "far advanced." Among the patients who were discharged, 63 were "apparently arrested" (patients who had no symptoms of the disease for a period of at least two months), 209 "improved" (patients whose symptoms had lessened or abated but who still had bacilli in their sputum), and 340 "unimproved." Over the four-year period, 322 patients died (32 percent of the total admissions). According to these numbers, barely over a quarter of patients left in better shape than when they came in. The same report also provided another set of statistics for admissions, discharges, and deaths at Waverly Hills from August 31, 1914, to January 1, 1916, with separate numbers for the "hospital" (the hospital for advanced cases) and for the "sanatorium" (the pavilions, cottages, and other accommodations for early and moderate cases). During this sixteen-month period, 146

REPORT OF WAVERLY HILL SANATORIUM AND HOSPITAL FROM JULY 26, 1910, to SEPTEMBER 1, 1914.

Male	593	
Females	415	
		1,008
Black	251	
White	757	
		1,008
Sputum Positive	592	
Sputum Negative	248	
Sputum Not Examined	168	
		1,008

STAGES ON ADMISSION.

Incipient	143	
Moderately Advanced	190	
Far Advanced	635	
Doubtful	5	
Negative	5	
Not Examined	30	
		1,008

STAGES ON DISCHARGE.

Apparently Arrested	63	
Improved	209	
Unimproved	340	
Died	322	
Under Treatment	74	
		1,008

AGES AND STAGES ON ADMISSION.

Ages	Incipient	Mod. Advanced	Far Advanced	
1 to 5	6	1	1	
5 to 10	34	11	7	
10 to 20	56	27	85	
20 to 30	26	66	180	
30 to 40	13	40	170	
40 to 50	6	28	108	
50 to 60	2	13	57	
60 to 70	0	4	22	
70 to 80	0	0	5	
	143	190	635	968

According to these numbers, 63 percent of admissions to Waverly Hills from July 26, 1910, to August 31, 1914, were in the far advanced stage of tuberculosis, and 32 percent died at the institution. Report of the Board of Tuberculosis Hospital, *rare pamphlet 362.16 B662 1916, Filson Historical Society.*

patients were admitted to the sanatorium, and 4 of them died (3 percent of sanatorium admissions). In contrast, 566 patients were admitted to the hospital for advanced cases, and 185 of them died (33 percent of hospital admissions).

REPORT OF THE WAVERLY HILLS SANATORIUM AND HOSPITAL, AUGUST 31, 1914–JANUARY 1, 1916

	Total Admissions	Left Against Medical Advice	Transferred to Hospital	Transferred to Sanatorium	Died	Deaths as Percentage of Patients Admitted
Sanatorium	146	78	25		4	3%
Hospital for advanced cases	566	238		126	185	33%

Source: Report of the Board Tuberculosis Hospital, *rare pamphlet 362.16 B662 1916, Filson Historical Society.*

A 1924 survey of hospitals in Louisville referred to deaths at Waverly Hills in the early 1920s as "numbering something less than 100 annually." The report presented specific patient numbers only for the year 1923, when 482 patients were treated at Waverly Hills (297 had been admitted that year, and the rest carried over from the previous year). Of that total, 91 patients (19 percent of the total number treated) died there. This decrease in the percentage of deaths at Waverly Hills from the mid-1910s is explained in large part by a significant increase in the number of "incipient" cases admitted to Waverly Hills, from 6 percent of admissions in 1913 to 29 percent in 1923. Incipient cases generally referred to individuals who had tested positive or who were suspected of having a bacterial infection but had not yet developed symptoms of tuberculosis. As we saw earlier in this book, many of the children admitted to Waverly Hills in these years, sometimes by order of the courts, had been exposed to a parent with an active case of tuberculosis but did not themselves show signs of the disease.[222]

Death certificates and Board of Health records help fill out information about the number of deaths at Waverly Hills Sanatorium for many years of its existence, as can be seen in the following table. Researchers John and Angela Amerine have sifted through all Jefferson County death certificates from certain years to compile individual and aggregate data about patients who died at Waverly Hills, information that John Amerine generously shared with me and gave me permission to cite.[223] For the years from 1943 to 1960, Board of Health reports list the total number of patients treated and the total number of deaths at Waverly Hills. According to the Amerines' research and Board of Health reports, the number of deaths at Waverly Hills reached a high of 162 in 1945 (18 percent of the total number of 903 patients treated).

By 1951, the number of deaths had decreased to 107 (14 percent of the total number of 743 patients treated). After this point, the number of deaths at the institution remained below 100 a year, with 53 deaths recorded in the fiscal year 1959–60 (8 percent of the total number of 684 patients treated).[224]

Number of Deaths at Waverly Hills Sanatorium, 1911–15, 1923, 1926–40, 1943–60

Year	Recorded Deaths
1911	30
1912	112
1913	114
1914	116
1915	141
1923	91
1926	73
1927	121
1928	88
1929	125
1930	104
1931	114
1932	96
1933	116
1934	121
1935	91
1936	93
1939	83
1940	106
1943	115
1944	146
1945	162
1946	161
1947	116
1948	107
1949	104

Year	Recorded Deaths
1950	88
1951	107
1952	79
1953	65
1954–55 fiscal year	42
1955–56 fiscal year	50
1956–57 fiscal year	65
1957–58 fiscal year	41
1958–59 fiscal year	50
1959–60 fiscal year	53
Total	**3,486**

Sources: John and Angela Amerine's survey of death certificates, 1911–15, 1926–36, 1939–40, 1946, and 1950–53; Haven Emerson and Anna C. Phillips, Hospitals and Health Agencies of Louisville 1924: A Survey, *48; Louisville and Jefferson County Board of Health, 1944–52, 1956–57 annual reports, 1954–60 statistical reports; "Health Board Will Offer Proposals for the Future of Waverly Hills,"* Courier-Journal, *December 4, 1955.*

These numbers, documenting nearly three-fourths of Waverly Hills Sanatorium's history, add up to almost 3,500 deaths. They include two particularly difficult periods—the early years of Waverly Hills and the years of World War II—when the institution's different facilities were caring for a high number of patients with advanced cases of tuberculosis and before the development of effective multidrug treatments. These numbers represent the very real and very painful experiences of thousands of patients who died at Waverly Hills, usually without loved ones by their side. They show how Waverly Hills Sanatorium, as a public institution committed to the aim of lowering rates of tuberculosis, took on the risk and care of high numbers of patients with advanced cases. The changing number of deaths over time highlights how patients faced very different levels of hope for recovery depending on the stage of their disease and the years they were treated.

Newspapers and obituaries help fill out the individual lives and stories behind the deaths at Waverly Hills. Many of the patients documented in the *Louisville Leader* were young. In 1923, "Little Ella Powell" died at the age of thirteen at Waverly Hills. She was a member of the Chestnut Street CME Church, and her funeral was led by Reverend D.L. Bayliss at the family's home at 912 West Madison Street. On October 20, 1928, the newspaper announced that "Miss Lucy Mosby," the twenty-one-year-old daughter of Mr. and Mrs. John Mosby, was seriously ill at Waverly Hills. She died just two and a half weeks later on November 7. In 1931, a woman expressed gratitude for "our neighbors and friends for the kindness shown us during the illness and death of our brother, Lee Andrew France," and for flowers sent by Dr. Orville Ballard and Esther Barrens from Waverly Hills. France had worked as a porter before contracting pulmonary tuberculosis and seeking treatment at Waverly Hills, where he died at the age of twenty-two.[225]

The *Courier-Journal* provided similarly tragic vignettes about individuals, such as an obituary for Emma Priddy, a thirty-four-year-old patient with a husband and eight children. Priddy died at Waverly Hills in 1926. A suicide death documented by the *Courier-Journal* and loosely related to Waverly Hills Sanatorium was that of William B. Harold, a sixty-six-year-old man who died after drinking poison at his home in 1921. "Mr. Harold had been in ill health for a year," the article reported, and in a despondent state. He died from suicide the same afternoon he "was to have been taken to Waverly Hills Sanatorium."[226]

One of the most frequently repeated anecdotes about deaths at Waverly Hills describes the staff's use of the main sanatorium's steam and supply tunnel to transport the bodies of those who died to an ambulance or hearse at the bottom of the hill. Evidence for this information seems to be primarily hearsay, but some of the sources include people who worked at Waverly Hills. The tunnel, which still exists today, was built to carry steam and to transport supplies by cable car from the main sanatorium down to the heating plant at the bottom of the hill. Dr. J. Frank W. Stewart wrote that "some time" before he joined the Waverly Hills medical staff in 1945, "the story goes that they would put the corpse on the cable car and let it down to the heating plant, where the ambulance would pick it up without the patients ever knowing that anyone had died." At one point, he had been told, the cable car carrying a body broke loose and crashed through the door at the bottom of the tunnel. "News got out about this happening," he wrote (though the *Courier-Journal* evidently did not cover the incident), "and that was the last of taking a corpse down through the tunnel."[227] The stories told to Dr. Stewart suggest that the tunnel was used to transport bodies for a limited span of time sometime after the opening of the main sanatorium in 1926 and before World War II. Decades later in 1986, a *Courier-Journal* article used the term *death tunnel* and attributed the idea to Waverly Hills board members, who in the late 1920s and 1930s would have been members of the Board of Tuberculosis Hospital.[228]

Administrators and staff throughout the history of Waverly Hills aimed to limit patients' exposure to deaths that occurred at the institution, while also handling the logistics and public repercussions of those deaths. In the 1910s and early 1920s, this was a near-impossible feat at the hospital for patients with advanced cases. "There is no room to isolate patients, and in fact the building is so crowded that we have no place for patients to die," said Board of Tuberculosis Hospital president A.H. Bowman in 1922, as he made a case for the funding and construction of a new sanatorium building. Unlike the pavilions and the hospital for advanced cases (which was converted into the Black hospital), the main sanatorium that opened in 1926 provided semiprivate rooms that helped shield many patients from the suffering and deaths of other patients. As Margaret Baugh recalled from her time at Waverly Hills in 1950 and 1951, staff would put a "do not disturb" sign on the doors of the rooms of patients who died. "You didn't know what happened to them," she said.[229]

Newspaper accounts and administrative records point to other grim parts of Waverly Hills Sanatorium's history. One dramatic tale involved Arthur Leo Barr, a thirty-four-year-old member of a prominent family from Pittsburgh, Pennsylvania, who ended up at Waverly Hills Sanatorium in 1912. The *Courier-Journal* described him as an artist "of a roving disposition and had refused to give the name of any relative or friend when received at the hospital." When he died in July at Waverly Hills, his body was turned over to the medical department at the University of Louisville for dissection, "as is customary in cases where a body is not claimed by relatives or friends within a month after death." Barr's family, with the help of a local detective and city health department officer Dr. W. Ed Grant, managed to track down Barr's body in a "pickling vat" at the medical school's morgue, "where it was found in a good state of preservation."[230]

Decades later, Board of Health meeting minutes from 1955 described a plan for the University of Louisville School of Medicine to send bodies used for dissection to a plot of Waverly Hills land for burial. At the Board of Health's monthly meeting on May 19, health department director Dr. C. Howe Eller explained to the board that the medical school's anatomy department had long used a plot in the West End of Louisville to bury the remains of the bodies used for dissection. Now the city wanted to move the bodies and use the land for other purposes. The medical school asked Dr. Eller to investigate whether a plot of unused Waverly Hills land could be used for burial. Dr. Eller told the board that carrying out the plan would require clandestine record keeping. One problem, he said, was that once a piece of land was used for the burial of human bodies, it could not be sold or used for any other purpose until the bodies were removed. Superintendent S.A. Ruskjer discussed a "remote area" about an acre in size on the Waverly Hills property that he thought would work, as long as no markers were used that "would interfere with the possible future sale of the adjoining area." After a "quite lengthy discussion" (the meeting minutes did not record any of the details of this part of the discussion), the following motion was unanimously carried: "Be it resolved by the Louisville and Jefferson County Board of Health that it hereby authorizes Mr. Ruskjer to designate a plot of ground on Waverly Hills Sanatorium property to be used by the Department of Anatomy of the Medical School for the burial of bodies used for dissection purposes."[231]

The *Courier-Journal* reported on the board meeting, as it did every month, but its coverage included no mention of the decision to bury bodies on the Waverly Hills grounds.[232] No mention of the proposal was made in subsequent board minutes, so it is not clear whether the plan was ever implemented. The board's post-meeting secrecy indicates that dissection remained a sensitive issue in the mid-twentieth century, decades after it was legalized in Kentucky in the late 1800s. Well into the twentieth century, the bodies of financially destitute individuals made up the vast majority of those used for medical training and typically included disproportionate numbers of African Americans. In Louisville, when individuals died at city or county public institutions and no family or friends claimed their bodies within three days, the bodies were given to the University of Louisville Medical School. The bodies were preserved from a month to a year to give families a chance to claim them, before being used for anatomical study. Kentucky law required physicians and medical schools to provide for the burial of the bodies. In 1955, the Board of Health and the medical school evidently intended to follow the law while also trying to hide their logistical plans for the burial of bodies from public view.[233]

The Board of Health plan highlights how Waverly Hills Sanatorium was part of a much bigger public health infrastructure and broader management of disease and death. Louisville and Jefferson County's anti-tuberculosis work involved various public agencies and private organizations, educational campaigns and legislation, schools and training programs, and state and federal funding. These entities and efforts aimed to lower rates of tuberculosis and provide diagnosis and treatment to those in need. They also built on fears about contagion and the "laboring masses" and perpetuated racial disparities in public services. The most troubling parts of Waverly Hills Sanatorium's history reveal how many individuals were not just dealing with the awful toll of tuberculosis but also grappling with blatant racial discrimination, poverty and financial insecurity, and separation from loved ones.

It is important to recognize how many people struggled and actively fought against those harsh realities, leaving a legacy of growth and change at Waverly Hills Sanatorium. The enormous number of people who sustained the institution over its half century of history included local residents and taxpayers, public officials, members of charitable associations, journalists, medical staff and employees, and patients willing to seek treatment there. They included those who wanted to protect the health of themselves and the general public. They included individuals who pushed for improvements and structural changes at Waverly Hills, lobbying for new facilities, demanding positions for Black physicians and nurses, and expanding educational and occupational programs for all patients. They included people who worked there because they had recovered from tuberculosis and those who never had tuberculosis but took on the risks of caring for patients with the disease. They included patients who left their homes and their families to spend months and years sharing a semiprivate room or a crowded ward with other patients. They included those who smuggled in liquor, who arranged card games and illegal betting, who formed friendships with others or learned to play a ukulele on their own, who underwent sputum tests and X-rays and surgical procedures, and who took part in the development of more effective treatments for tuberculosis. Because of these varied forms of treatment and support, there were patients who were able to persevere, improve their health, and leave the sanatorium to live long lives.

History is an ongoing process of investigation, and there are many more stories to uncover and tell about the sprawling complex of Waverly Hills Sanatorium and its patients and staff. Tuberculosis, moreover, is not a bygone disease. Due in large part to multidrug-resistant strains, tuberculosis remains a leading cause of death among infectious diseases worldwide, ranking behind only COVID-19 in 2020.[234] Indeed, as we continue to navigate daunting public health challenges, as all kinds of workers help to provide and care for others, and as many people take daily precautions to help protect themselves and the most vulnerable in our society, it is possible to look back to the history of Waverly Hills Sanatorium and see a past bearing important similarities to our own time.

NOTES

Introduction

1. "Waverly Hills," *Courier-Journal*, August 23, 1983; "Design for Massive Jesus Statue Unveiled; Gender, Race Blurred," *Courier-Journal*, September 20, 1996; "Historic Hospital Could Be Torn Down," *Courier-Journal*, March 10, 2001; "Owners Saving Sanatorium," *Courier-Journal*, Dec. 20, 2006, 3. All clippings in reference file on Health: Waverly Hills, University of Louisville Archives and Special Collections [ULASC].
2. Edward Arthur Waverly Hills Photograph Collection, 019PC9, Filson Historical Society [FHS]; 1920 United States federal census, death certificate for Edwin [*sic*] A. Arthur, ancestry.com.
3. Email from David Price, president of Waverly Hills Historical Society, May 12, 2020.
4. A transcribed and fully searchable version of the collection is available on the University of Louisville Archives and Special Collections website, digital.library.louisville.edu/cdm/description/collection/leader.
5. "Esther Maxwell Barrens," nkaa.uky.edu/nkaa/items/show/790; 1930 United States federal census, ancestry.com; "Crowned: Miss Marie Barrens," *Louisville Leader*, October 24, 1931.

Chapter 1

6. Helen Bynum, *Spitting Blood: The History of Tuberculosis* (Oxford: Oxford University Press, 2015), xiv–xxiii; "Tuberculosis, Like Covid, Spreads by Breathing, Scientists Report," *New York Times*, October 19, 2021.

7. Sheila Rothman, *Living in the Shadow of Death: Tuberculosis and the Social Experience of Illness in American History* (Baltimore: Johns Hopkins University Press, 1994), 2–6, 14–17, 132; Katherine Ott, *Fevered Lives: Tuberculosis in American Culture since 1870* (Cambridge, MA: Harvard University Press, 1996), 9–13; "Children Call for Quick Aid," *Courier-Journal*, October 31, 1915, A2.
8. William A. M'Dowell, MD, *Reply of William A. M'Dowell to Dr. Yandell's Rejoinder, in a Controversy Relative to Cure of Consumption* (Louisville, KY: Prentice and Weissinger, 1844), rare pamphlet 619.995 M138 1844, FHS; Ott, *Fevered Lives*, 27.
9. February–April 1853 letters, folder 9, Brown-Ewell Family Papers, Mss. A B877a, FHS; D.J. Haggard to Martha A. Adams, December 19, 1858, Martha Adams Papers, Mss. C A, FHS; Ann W. Beatty to Sarah Beatty, October 20, 1849, folder 79, Beatty-Quisenberry Family Papers, Mss. A B369, FHS; Rothman, *Living in the Shadow of Death*, 16–17; Bynum, *Spitting Blood*, xiv–xxiii.
10. Rothman, *Living in the Shadow of Death*, 2; Bynum, *Spitting Blood*, 77–78; Agatha Logan Marshall to cousin Tom, June 6, 1873, folder 549, Bullitt Family Papers—Oxmoor collection, Mss. A B937c, FHS; James C. Stewart to Arba Hardy, February 11, 1850, folder 3, Hiram Wingate Papers, Mss. A W769, FHS.
11. Bynum, *Spitting Blood*, 69–81; Charles Rosenberg, *The Care of Strangers: The Rise of America's Hospital System* (Baltimore: Johns Hopkins University Press, 1987), chs. 1–4.
12. O.H.P. Anderson to Orlando Brown, December 21, 1842, folder 39, Orlando Brown Papers, Mss. A B879, FHS.
13. Oliver Hazard Perry Anderson to Henry Wingate, January 12, 1843, Mss. C A, FHS.
14. William L. Allen to Young E. Allison, October 12, 1902, Young Ewing Allison Papers, Mss. A A439a, FHS; Bynum, *Spitting Blood*, 82–85, 132–39; Rothman, *Living in the Shadow of Death*, 136–72, 201–26.
15. Bynum, *Spitting Blood*, 95-123; Rothman, *Living in the Shadow of Death*, 179-83.
16. Rothman, *Living in the Shadow of Death*, 198.

Chapter 2

17. John E. Kleber, ed., *The Encyclopedia of Louisville* (Lexington: University Press of Kentucky, 2000), 18.
18. City of Louisville, *Annual Reports for the Fiscal Year Ending August 31, 1903, and December 31, 1903* (Louisville, KY: Courier-Journal Job Printing, 1905), 519; *Proceedings of the First Annual Meeting of the Kentucky Anti-Tuberculosis Association*, January 8, 1906, pamphlet 614.542 K37, FHS.

19. *Report of the Board of Tuberculosis Hospital, 1906–1915*, 43, rare pamphlet 362.16 B662 1916, FHS; "Waverly Hills Was Financed by City, County," *Courier-Journal*, July 24, 1960, 63.
20. *Proceedings of the First Annual Meeting of the Kentucky Anti-Tuberculosis Association*, 1, 3.
21. "Changes Name and Hears Many Reports," *Courier-Journal*, February 12, 1909, 4; "Scope Widens…Annual Meeting of Anti-Tuberculosis Association," *Courier-Journal*, April 12, 1910, 4; *34th Annual Report of the Louisville Tuberculosis Association*, 1938, 27, pamphlet 614.542 L888, FHS; "April 25 Designated as Tuberculosis Day," *Courier-Journal*, April 6, 1911, 3.
22. *Proceedings of the First Annual Meeting of the Kentucky Anti-Tuberculosis Association*, 4; *34th Annual Report of the Louisville Tuberculosis Association*; Rothman, *Living in the Shadow of Death*, 184.
23. Rothman, *Living in the Shadow of Death*, 184–86.
24. *Six Years' Work in Louisville* (Louisville, KY, 1911), 3, vol. 4, Louisville Tuberculosis Association (formerly Louisville Anti-Tuberculosis Assn.) Minutes, 1912–19, Mss. BA L888a, FHS; Nancy Tomes, *The Gospel of Germs: Men, Women and the Microbe in American Life* (Cambridge, MA: Harvard University Press, 1998).
25. Temple Bodley, undated speech, folder 159, 1907 speech, folder 156, Bodley family papers, Mss. A B668e, FHS.
26. Temple Bodley, *A War upon Consumption: An Appeal to the Women of Louisville to Help Drive the Disease from the City*, 1905, Kentucky Anti-Tuberculosis Association, Louisville, KY, folder 159, Bodley family papers.
27. Bodley, 1907 speech; Bodley, *War upon Consumption.*
28. *Bulletin*, December 1929, 5, vol. 78, Louisville Women's City Club records, 1917–85, Mss. BM L888; "Prevention of Consumption," *Messenger-Inquirer* (Owensboro, KY), July 5, 1908, 4.
29. City of Louisville, *Annual Reports for the Fiscal Year Ending August 31, 1903, and December 31, 1903*, 521–22.
30. City of Louisville, *Annual Reports for the Fiscal Year Ending August 31, 1911 and December 31, 1911* (Louisville, KY: Geo. G. Fetter, 1911), 412–13, FHS; Mary K. Marlatt, "Progressive City in the Progressive Era: Child Welfare Reform in Louisville Kentucky," University of Louisville master's thesis, 2019, 55–68, doi.org/10.18297/etd/3176.
31. "First of Year: Tuberculosis Hospital Board Will Be Named," *Courier-Journal*, December 26, 1906, 8; *Six Years' Work in Louisville*, 9; City of Louisville, *Annual Reports for the Fiscal Year Ending August 31, 1911 and December 31, 1911*, 399; National Association for the Study and Prevention of Tuberculosis, *A Tuberculosis Directory Containing a List of Institutions, Associations and Other Agencies Dealing with Tuberculosis in the United States and*

Canada (New York, 1911), 228, babel.hathitrust.org; "Timely Words by the Health Officer," *Courier-Journal*, October 31, 1928.

32. City of Louisville, *Annual Reports for the Fiscal Year Ending August 31, 1903, and December 31, 1903*, 519; City of Louisville, *Annual Reports for the Fiscal Year Ending August 31, 1906 and December 31, 1906* (Louisville, KY: Globe Printing, 1907), 430; Tera W. Hunter, *To 'Joy My Freedom: Southern Black Women's Lives and Labors after the Civil War* (Cambridge, MA: Harvard University Press, 1997), 187–218; George Wright, *Life Behind the Veil: Blacks in Louisville, Kentucky, 1865–1930* (Baton Rouge: Louisiana State University Press, 1985), 78–122.

33. Haven Emerson and Anna C. Phillips, *Hospitals and Health Agencies of Louisville 1924: A Survey*, made for the Health and Hospital Survey Committee of the Louisville Community Chest, 3, 41–42, babel.hathitrust.org.

34. *Bulletin*, July 1924, vol. 78, minutes, May 5, 1924, folder 13, Louisville Women's City Club records; Gail Elizabeth Chooljian Nall, "Louise C. Morel, the Louisville Women's City Club, and Municipal Housekeeping in Louisville, 1917–1935," University of Louisville master's thesis, 2004, 63–69, ir.library.louisville.edu/cgi/viewcontent.cgi?article=2037&context=etd.

35. Health Committee minutes, November 10, November 17, 1922, folder 32, Louisville Women's City Club records.

36. "Renewed Energy Infused into Anti-Tuberculosis Movement," *Courier-Journal*, March 19, 1906; "Mayor Makes Appointments," *Courier-Journal*, December 29, 1906, 2; "First of Year: Tuberculosis Hospital Board Will Be Named," *Courier-Journal*, December 26, 1906, 8; "Waverly Hills Was Financed by City, County," *Courier-Journal*, July 24, 1960, 63.

37. "History of Waverly Hills Sanatorium," possibly written by Catherine Richardson, circa 1955, 2–3, Kornhauser Health Sciences Library, University of Louisville [Kornhauser]; *Report of the Board of Tuberculosis Hospital, 1906–1915*, 48.

38. "To Teach Hygiene: Tuberculosis Dispensary Is Now Being Conducted," *Courier-Journal*, November 23, 1908, 3; *Report of the Board of Tuberculosis Hospital, 1906–1915*, 50.

39. *Six Years' Work in Louisville*, 4, 14; City of Louisville, *Annual Reports for the Fiscal Year Ending August 31, 1910 and December 31, 1910* (Louisville, KY: Geo. G. Fetter Company, 1910), 838, FHS.

40. Louisville Anti-Tuberculosis Association, *The Hazelwood Sanatorium* (Louisville, KY, circa 1917), 10, rare pamphlet 362.16 H429, FHS.

41. Louisville Anti-Tuberculosis Association, *Hazelwood Sanatorium*; "Report of Physician in Charge of Hazelwood Sanatorium," March 31, 1917, vol. 2, Louisville Tuberculosis Association (formerly Louisville Anti-Tuberculosis

Assn.) Minutes, 1912–19; *Reports of Officers of the Association Sanatorium, to the Annual Meeting of Its Members, May 17, 1910*, 10, rare pamphlet 362.196995 A849 1910, FHS; April 1916 minutes, vol. 1, Louisville Tuberculosis Association, 1911–19 (formerly Louisville Anti-Tuberculosis Assn.) Minutes.

42. City of Louisville, *Annual Reports for the Fiscal Year Ending August 31, 1912 and December 31, 1912* (Louisville, KY: Geo. G. Fetter Company), 504, FHS; Louisville Anti-Tuberculosis Association, *Hazelwood Sanatorium*, 10.

Chapter 3

43. "Action to Be Taken at Once: Temporary Building to Be Erected at Hospital for Isolation of Persons with Tuberculosis," *Courier-Journal*, August 13, 1906, 1.

44. "Plans Ready: Mayor Has Drawings for Tuberculosis Hospital," *Courier-Journal*, October 23, 1906, 10; "First of Year: Tuberculosis Hospital Board Will Be Named," *Courier-Journal*, December 26, 1906, 8.

45. "Tuberculosis Hospital Site Formally Transferred," *Courier-Journal*, January 22, 1908, 5; letter to Tom Owen from Catharine Own Ellis, October 20, 2001, reference file on Health: Waverly Hills; Bodley, 1907 speech; "Tuberculosis Hospital Board on Site Contention," *Courier-Journal*, February 4, 1908, 4.

46. "Its Jurisdiction: Board of Health Uncertain and Defers Action," *Courier-Journal*, January 31, 1908; "Retreat That Board of Tuberculosis Hospital Will Build at Waverly Hill," *Courier-Journal*, November 15, 1908, A7; "Tuberculosis Hospital Board on Site Contention," *Courier-Journal*, February 4, 1908, 4; Martin E. Biemer, James B. Calvert, and George H. Yater, *Louisville's Street Railways and How They Shaped the City's Growth* (Louisville, KY: Butler Books, 2018), 81–95.

47. "Retreat That Board of Tuberculosis Hospital Will Build at Waverly Hill," *Courier-Journal*, November 15, 1908, A7; "Well Pleased with Grounds and Buildings," *Courier-Journal*, March 9, 1910, 14; City of Louisville, *Annual Reports for the Fiscal Year Ending August 31, 1910 and December 31, 1910*, 837; "History of Waverly Hills Sanatorium," 2.

48. "History of Waverly Hills Sanatorium," 1; "Opening of Waverly Hill Sanatorium," *Courier-Journal*, October 2, 1910, A3; "Dedicated to the Cause of Humanity: Anti-Tuberculosis Hospital Opened at Waverly," *Courier-Journal*, October 13, 1910, 12.

49. *Report of the Board of Tuberculosis Hospital, 1906–1915*, 6, 30.

50. "Scope Widens…Annual Meeting of Anti-Tuberculosis Association," *Courier-Journal*, April 12, 1910, 4; "White Plague Causes Scrap," *Courier-Journal*, March 31, 1911, 6.

51. "$25,000 for Care of Tuberculosis Patients," *Courier-Journal*, April 18, 1911, 5; "In Special Car: Tubercular Patients to Be Taken to Waverly Hill," *Courier-Journal*, August 22, 1911, 5; "Unique Colony of Plague Convalescents among Forest-Hooded Hills," *Courier-Journal*, August 27, 1911, C12; *Report of the Board of Tuberculosis Hospital, 1906–1915*, 30.
52. JF 75-76 Waverly Hills Tuberculosis Sanitarium 8101 Dixie Highway, folder: Waverly Hills Tuberculosis Sanitarium, J.J. Gaffney 1909, Arthur Loomis, arch., 1922–1926, Samuel W. Thomas papers, 2012_020-PA, ULASC.
53. "Louisville: Cures Not Dream, Born of Enthusiasm," *Courier-Journal*, March 25, 1913, B9.
54. "History of Waverly Hills Sanatorium," 3–4; *Report of the Board of Tuberculosis Hospital, 1906–1915*, 33–34; *Reports of Officers of the Association Sanatorium, to the Annual Meeting of Its Members, May 17, 1910*, 12.
55. "Children Call for Quick Aid," *Courier-Journal*, October 31, 1915, A2; "Urge Need of Waverly Children's Pavilion," *Courier-Journal*, November 19, 1915, 5; "Waverly Superintendent Favors Increased Levy," *Courier-Journal*, October 15, 1915, 10.
56. "Plan Musicale for Benefit of Sanatorium Patients," *Courier-Journal*, December 27, 1911, 5; "Theory Happily Proved in Open Air School," *Courier-Journal*, April 28, 1912, C1.
57. "Theory Happily Proved in Open Air School," *Courier-Journal*, April 28, 1912, C1.
58. *Report of the Board of Tuberculosis Hospital, 1906–1915*, 12; "Waverly Hill Children's Carnival Next Saturday," *Courier-Journal*, June 27, 1915, 10; "Welfare Notes," *Courier-Journal*, April 30, 1916, A11; "Sanatorium School Support," *Courier-Journal*, October 27, 1922, 4; "History of Waverly Hills Sanatorium," 12.
59. "$1,000,000 for Hospital Urged," *Courier-Journal*, January 1, 1922, 5; Richard Allen Heckman and Betty Jean Hall, "Berea College and the Day Law," *Register of the Kentucky Historical Society* 66 (January 1968): 35–52.
60. "Welfare Notes," *Courier-Journal*, March 5, 1916, A10; "Fighting for Health at Waverly Hills," *Courier-Journal*, January 9, 1921, 57.
61. National Association for the Study and Prevention of Tuberculosis, *A Tuberculosis Directory Containing a List of Institutions, Associations and Other Agencies Dealing with Tuberculosis in the United States and Canada* (New York, 1916), 27, babel.hathitrust.org.
62. "Unique Colony of Plague Convalescents among Forest-Hooded Hills," *Courier-Journal*, August 27, 1911, C12.
63. Ibid.; City of Louisville, *Annual Reports for the Fiscal Year Ending August 31, 1912 and December 31, 1912*, 504.

64. *Report of the Board of Tuberculosis Hospital, 1906–1915*, 17; "Unique Colony of Plague Convalescents among Forest-Hooded Hills," *Courier-Journal*, August 27, 1911, C12; "Children Call for Quick Aid," *Courier-Journal*, October 31, 1915, A2.
65. "Fighting for Health at Waverly Hills," *Courier-Journal*, January 9, 1921, 57; B.S. Herben, MD, "Light in the Treatment of Tuberculosis," *St. Matthews Booster*, October 20, 1927, vol. 2, scrapbooks containing publicity pertaining to TB health facilities (esp. Waverly Hills Sanatorium)…By Louisville Tuberculosis Association, SB L888, FHS; Bynum, *Spitting Blood*, 152–53.
66. "Dedicated to the Cause of Humanity: Anti-Tuberculosis Hospital Opened at Waverly," *Courier-Journal*, October 13, 1910, 12; "Two Nurses to Compose First Graduating Class: School of Tuberculosis Hospital Will Have Commencement Next Fall," *Courier-Journal*, March 18, 1912, 10; "Three Young Nurses Are Given Diplomas," *Courier-Journal*, November 10, 1912, B1; "Fighting for Health at Waverly Hills," *Courier-Journal*, January 9, 1921, 57.
67. "Denies Wilson Asked to Quit," *Courier-Journal*, August 1, 1916, 5; "Dr. J.B. Floyd Elected Head of Waverly Hill," *Courier-Journal*, September 18, 1916, 2; May 29, 1918 minutes, vol. 2, Louisville Tuberculosis Association (formerly Louisville Anti-Tuberculosis Assn.) Minutes.
68. University of Michigan Center for the History of Medicine, "The American Influenza Epidemic of 1918–1919: Louisville, Kentucky," Influenza Encyclopedia, www.influenzaarchive.org/cities/city-louisville.html.
69. *Tonics and Sedatives* (Louisville, KY: Louisville City Hospital Training School for Nurses, 1919), 29–30, Kornhauser; "Waverly Hills Training School," March 1942, folder: List of Grads and Curriculum and History, Waverly Hills Training School for Nurses, Record Group 194, Kornhauser.
70. "Opera, Jazz and Ice Cream Cheer Veterans at Waverly Hills," *Courier-Journal*, August 21, 1921, 3; "Fighting for Health at Waverly Hills," *Courier-Journal*, January 9, 1921, 57.

Chapter 4

71. Emerson and Phillips, *Hospitals and Health Agencies of Louisville 1924*, 51–52; "Hospital to Be Started May 12," *Courier-Journal*, April 20, 1924, 60; "Plan to Finance Hospital Drawn," *Courier-Journal*, January 4, 1922, 5.
72. "$1,000,000 for Hospital Urged," *Courier-Journal*, January 1, 1922, 5; "Plan to Finance Hospital Drawn," *Courier-Journal*, January 4, 1922, 5; "Jury Scores Dry Holdups," *Courier Journal*, April 29, 1922, 1.
73. "Air Circus Plans Are Completed," *Courier-Journal*, May 28, 1922, 10; "City Club Will Manage Sales for Benefit of Waverly Hills Sanatorium,"

Courier-Journal, June 11, 1922, B3; "Elks Pay Honor to Dead Airmen," *Courier-Journal*, June 26, 1922, 12.

74. *Courier-Journal*, October 30, 1922, 12.
75. "Let's Make It a Better Louisville, a Greater Louisville," advertisement, *Courier-Journal*, November 5, 1922, A2.
76. "Memorial and Hospital Bond Issues Carry," *Courier-Journal*, November 8, 1922, 1; "Loomis Selected to Draw Plans for T.B. Hospital," *Louisville Times*, November 22, 1922, newspaper clipping, and JF75-76 Waverly Hills Sanitarium 8101 Dixie Highway, folder: Waverly Hills Tuberculosis Sanitarium, Samuel W. Thomas papers; "Hospital to Be Started May 12," *Courier-Journal*, April 20, 1924, 60; "Earth Turned at Waverly," *Courier-Journal*, May 13, 1924, 1.
77. "History of Waverly Hills Sanatorium," 2.
78. "New Sanatorium Here Dedicated," *Courier-Journal*, October 21, 1926, 1, 3; "Building at Waverly Hills Complete," *Jeffersonian*, September 9, 1926, and "Hospital to Be Dedicated Oct. 20," *Louisville Times*, October 7, 1926, scrapbooks containing publicity pertaining to TB health facilities (esp. Waverly Hills Sanatorium)...by Louisville Tuberculosis Association.
79. "Crowd to See Dedication of New Hospital," *Courier-Journal*, October 17, 1926; "New Sanatorium Here Dedicated," *Courier-Journal*, October 21, 1926, 1, 3.
80. "History of Waverly Hills Sanatorium," 8, 17.
81. Luther Adams, *Way Up North in Louisville: African American Migration in the Urban South, 1930–1970* (Chapel Hill: University of North Carolina Press, 2010), ch. 2.
82. Archibald C. McIntyre, "The Colored Department at Waverly Hill," The Point of View, *Courier-Journal*, June 30, 1928, 6.
83. Emerson and Phillips, *Hospitals and Health Agencies of Louisville 1924*, 65, 90; "Inter-Racial Commission Announces Program," *Louisville Leader*, May 16, 1925.
84. "History of Waverly Hills Sanatorium," 6; *Waverly Herald*, May–June 1955, vol. IV–1, Kornhauser.
85. "History of Waverly Hills Sanatorium," 6, 9, 11.
86. *Louisville Leader*, July 21, 1928; McIntyre, "Colored Department at Waverly Hill," 6; "Tubercular Clinic at Sunshine Center" [unidentified newspaper], January 31, 1927, scrapbooks containing publicity pertaining to TB health facilities (esp. Waverly Hills Sanatorium)...by Louisville Tuberculosis Association; "History of Waverly Hills Sanatorium," 10.
87. *Louisville Leader*, July 21, 1928.
88. *Louisville Leader*, July 23, 1927; "History of Waverly Hills Sanatorium," 9.

89. 1920 United States federal census, 1922 city directory for Seymour, Indiana, ancestry.com; Merrill Montgomery to Lynn Faulkoner, Wednesday, August 3 [1927], undated, folder 4, box 1, Merrill Montgomery correspondence, 2011_063-UA, ULASC.
90. Montgomery to Faulkoner, Monday, December 1 [1927], folder 3, Merrill Montgomery correspondence.
91. Montgomery to Faulkoner, Monday [1928], Merrill Montgomery correspondence.
92. Montgomery to Faulkoner, Hazelwood State Sanitorium, Monday [late July or early August 1927], folder 3, Merrill Montgomery correspondence.
93. Montgomery to Faulkoner, Waverly Hills Sanatorium, Thursday, September 20, 1928, Merrill Montgomery correspondence.
94. "Hospital Bars Non-Residents," *Courier-Journal*, March 21, 1928, 26; "Waverly Hill Policy Given," *Courier-Journal*, October 27, 1929, 1–2.
95. Montgomery to Faulkoner, Waverly Hills Sanatorium, Thursday, September 20, 1928, Merrill Montgomery correspondence; Bynum, *Spitting Blood*, xxv.
96. "Out for 3 Months Instead of 26, Today's Tubercular Is in Luck," *Courier-Journal*, March 20, 1938, 66; Bynum, *Spitting Blood*, 152–59.
97. Montgomery to Faulkoner, Waverly Hills Sanatorium, Thursday, September 20, 1928, Merrill Montgomery correspondence.
98. Death certificate for Merrill M. Montgomery, ancestry.com.
99. Stella Hatfield to "Miss Overman," February 6, 1929, folder 55, Robert Worth Bingham additional papers, Mss. A B613d, FHS.
100. Hatfield to Overman, February 6, March 4, April 14, August 8, August 27, October 3, November [no day, near Thanksgiving], 1929, folder 55, Bingham additional papers.
101. Hatfield to Overman, March 4, March 18, April 14, May 1, May 28, 1929, folder 55, Bingham additional papers.
102. Hatfield to Overman, March 4, May 28, November 2, 1929, folder 55, Bingham additional papers; "Work Aids Mental and Physical Ill of Louisville and State in Occupational Therapy Classes," *Courier-Journal*, May 6, 1923, 38; "Exhibit of Articles Made by Waverly Hill Patients Opens," *Courier-Journal*, May 19, 1925, 20; "History of Waverly Hills Sanatorium," 9, 14.
103. Hatfield to Overman, July 1, 1930, folder 75, Bingham additional papers.
104. Hatfield to Ruth, October 12, 1930, folder 82, Bingham additional papers.
105. Alice Turner to Robert Bingham, October 14, 1930, folder 82, Bingham additional papers.

106. Hatfield to Overman, November 13, November 28, 1930, folder 75, Bingham additional papers.
107. Death certificate for Stella Hatfield, May 8, 1931, ancestry.com.

Chapter 5

108. "2,959 Names on City's Payroll," *Courier-Journal*, June 27, 1930, 24; "Post Office at Waverley Hills," *Courier-Journal*, April 24, 1931, 9; "Yours for Health," *Courier-Journal*, November 22, 1937, 6.
109. "Women Voters Visit Sanatorium," *Courier-Journal*, November 11, 1931, 7; "New Manager at Sanatorium," *Courier-Journal*, September 24, 1930, 10; "Tuberculosis Deaths Decline," *Courier-Journal*, June 16, 1934, 20; "You Can Have Tuberculosis without Symptoms," *Courier-Journal*, May 20, 1939, 38; "Waverley Hills Cuts Deficit to $31,000," *Courier-Journal*, June 21, 1940, 37.
110. "Laffoon Starts Rest at Waverly Hills," *Courier-Journal*, April 5, 1934, 1; "Laffoon Back at Capitol," *Courier-Journal*, April 18, 1934, 11.
111. *34th Annual Report of the Louisville Tuberculosis Association*, 3–5, 7; *Waverly Herald*, IV, issue 1 (May–June 1955), Kornhauser; *On the Firing Line*, www.c-span.org/video/?322245-1/1936-documentary-on-firing-line; "Yours for Health," *Courier-Journal*, November 22, 1937, 6; "Postural Idea Used in War on Tuberculosis," *Courier-Journal*, December. 9, 1938, 2.
112. Linda Hope Carew, "Along King's Highway," *Courier-Journal*, July 6, 1930, April 6, 1930, December 7, 1930, September 30, 1934, September 15, 1935, April 12, 1936.
113. "A Protest from Waverley Hills," *Courier-Journal*, May 4, 1932, 6.
114. *On the Firing Line*.
115. "Proceedings of Louisville and Jefferson County White House Conference on Child Health and Protection," April 26, 1932, 24–25, Kornhauser; *34th Annual Report of the Louisville Tuberculosis Association*, 3–5, 7; "You Can Have Tuberculosis without Symptoms," *Courier-Journal*, May 20, 1939, 38; "Students Hail X-Ray Test as Fun," *Courier-Journal*, December 11, 1927, 11; Frances Fanelli, "A Study of Forty-Three Patients Who Left Waverly Hills Sanatorium against the Doctor's Advice during the Period September 1 through December 31, 1942" (1944), 28, ir.library.louisville.edu/etd/1934.
116. "Millions Held Hospital Need," *Courier-Journal*, April 23, 1930, 1; "Maximum Levy Asked by Hospital," *Courier-Journal*, April 26, 1930, 3; "New Building Urged," *Courier-Journal*, July 4, 1930, 26; "Two Hospital Units Asked," *Courier-Journal*, August 9, 1930, 2.
117. "New Unit to Go Up at Waverley Hills," *Courier-Journal*, June 28, 1932, 2; *Louisville Leader*, March 4, March 11, 1933; "Report Lauds Record of

Waverley Hills," *Courier-Journal*, June 21, 1934, 8; "History of Waverly Hills Sanatorium," 10.

118. *Louisville Leader*, March 18, 1933.

119. Ibid., October 24, 1931; April 1, 1933; April 21, 1934; April 6, August 10, July 20, 1935; September 17, 1938; "Waverly Hills Nursing Chief Is Dead at 66," *Courier-Journal*, August 15, 1954, 25.

120. "Yule Parties Planned, *Courier-Journal*, December 22, 1929, 31; *Louisville Leader*, March 2, 1929; April 15, May 6, June 17, 1933; December 2, 1939.

121. "Magazines for Waverley Hills," *Courier-Journal*, April 15, 1934, 42.

122. "More Attractive City to Greet Visitors to Louisville This Year," *Courier-Journal*, May 4, 1938, 21; "History of Waverly Hills Sanatorium," 12; *Waverly Herald*, IV, issue 1 (May–June 1955); "Loudspeaker Curriculum Is Varied," *Courier-Journal*, March 6, 1937.

123. "1,500 Refugees Found Heat, Light and Water at Waverly," *Courier-Journal*, February 5, 1937, 7; "Births: Gus William and Eugenia W. Hinderer, Waverley Hills Sanitorium, Waverley Hills, Ky., Boy, January 27," *Courier-Journal*, February 19, 1937, 27.

Chapter 6

124. "Kentuckians at Camp Shelby to Get Furloughs during Holiday," *Courier-Journal*, November 16, 1941; "Tuberculosis in Louisville," Report of the Tuberculosis Committee of the Health Council, December 1942, 5–6, Kornhauser; Louisville and Jefferson County Health Department, 1942 annual report, 6, Kornhauser; Louisville and Jefferson County Health Department, 1944 annual report, 95; Fanelli, "Study of Forty-Three Patients Who Left Waverly Hills," 10.

125. "Radio Debate Staged on Waverley Merger," *Courier-Journal*, January 26, 1942, "Dr. Miller of Waverley Hills Attacks Consolidation Plan, Points to Lower Death Rate," *Courier-Journal*, January 26, 1942, "Senators Predict Passage of Bill Including Waverley in Merger," *Courier-Journal*, January 29, 1942, vol. 4, scrapbooks containing publicity pertaining to TB health facilities (esp. Waverly Hills Sanatorium)…by Louisville Tuberculosis Association; Letter to the Editor, *Courier-Journal*, January 30, 1942, 6.

126. "Senators Predict Passage of Bill Including Waverley in Merger," *Courier-Journal*, January 29, 1942; "Waverley Hills Should Not Be Exempted," *Courier-Journal*, January 23, 1942, vol. 4, scrapbooks containing publicity pertaining to TB health facilities (esp. Waverly Hills Sanatorium)…by Louisville Tuberculosis Association.

127. "The City Hospital and Waverley Hills," *Courier-Journal*, January 17, 1942; "Wyatt Says 'Politics' in Health Merger Is Only a Specter in

Opponents' Minds," *Courier-Journal*, January 29, 1942; "What Would We 'Save' Waverley From?," *Courier-Journal*, January 29, 1942, vol. 4, scrapbooks containing publicity pertaining to TB health facilities (esp. Waverly Hills Sanatorium)...by Louisville Tuberculosis Association.

128. "Senate Defeats Efforts to Ban Waverley Merger," *Courier-Journal*, January 30, 1942, 1, 21; Louisville and Jefferson County Board of Health, meeting minutes, March 19, 1942; "General Hospital Begins Its New Lease on Life Today," *Courier-Journal*, July 1, 1979, 1.

129. "On Again, Off Again," *Courier-Journal*, March 11, 1945, 52.

130. "W.P.B. Approves $165,000 Addition at Waverley Hills for Negroes," *Courier-Journal*, August 25, 1942; "Waverley Negro Wing a Satisfying Addition," *Courier-Journal*, August 27, 1942; "Ballard, Waverly Hills Honored by Howard University," *Courier-Journal*, February 25, 1943, 13; "Dedication at Waverley Set for Oct. 24," *Courier-Journal*, October 17, 1943, 54; Louisville and Jefferson County Health Department, 1943 annual report, 3, 1944 annual report, 99.

131. Louisville and Jefferson County Health Department, 1945 annual report, 94; "Ballard, Waverly Hills Honored by Howard University," *Courier-Journal*, February 25, 1943, 13; "Dedication at Waverley Set for Oct. 24," *Courier-Journal*, October 17, 1943, 54; *Louisville Leader*, February 27, 1943.

132. "Ruskjer Named Waverly Hills Superintendent," *Courier-Journal*, July 25, 1945, 11; Louisville and Jefferson County Health Department, 1945 annual report, 88.

133. "White Charges Drunkenness, Gaming, Politics at Waverly," *Courier-Journal*, September 22, 1945, 8.

134. "Waverly Patients—Some, Anyway—Miss Their 'Therapeutic' Betting," *Courier-Journal*, September 22, 1945, 8.

135. "Ruskjer Says County Police Took T.B. Patients to Polls," *Courier-Journal*, December 13, 1945; Louisville and Jefferson County Board of Health, meeting minutes, September 27, 1945; "2 Reports Say White Wrong about Waverly/Accusation of Bookmaking by Worker Is Only Charge Substantiated by Board," *Courier-Journal*, October 2, 1945, 9.

136. Louisville and Jefferson County Board of Health, meeting minutes, September 27, 1945; "2 Reports Say White Wrong about Waverly/Accusation of Bookmaking by Worker Is Only Charge Substantiated by Board," *Courier-Journal*, October 2, 1945, 9.

137. Report of a Committee of Five Members of the Jefferson County Medical Society Appointed by the President, Dr. M.C. Buckles, to Investigate Conditions at Waverly Hills Sanatorium, Louisville and Jefferson County Board of Health, meeting minutes, November 29, 1945;

"Doctors Give Waverly Hills Clean Bill," *Courier-Journal*, December 21, 1945, 1, 16.

138. "Waverly Hills Is Still a Model Institution," *Courier-Journal*, December 22, 1945, 6; "Defends Waverly Hills," *Courier-Journal*, October 7, 1945, 32; "Waverly Hills Advisory Board," *Courier-Journal*, November 7, 1945, 6; "Waverly Hills Praised Highly by Grand Jury," *Courier-Journal*, November 3, 1945, 13; "Grand Jury Raps Low Pay at Lakeland," *Courier-Journal*, December 22, 1945, 5.

139. "Waverly Staff Given Vote of Confidence," *Courier-Journal*, March 16, 1946, 4; "'Rotten Administrators' at Two Hospitals Charged," *Courier-Journal*, July 13, 1946, 4; "Praises Waverly Hills," *Courier-Journal*, January 21, 1948, 6.

140. Louisville and Jefferson County Board of Health, meeting minutes, August 9, 1945, monthly progress reports, December 1947, October 1949; "3 City and County Institutions' Farms Rake in Crops and Cash Surpluses," *Courier-Journal*, August 8, 1948, 12; "Hotels in City Threaten to Shut Dining Rooms," *Courier-Journal*, September 20, 1946, 1.

141. Louisville and Jefferson County Health Department, 1945 annual report, 88–89; "3 City and County Institutions' Farms Rake in Crops and Cash Surpluses," *Courier-Journal*, August 8, 1948, 12; "Waverly Hills Hogs Selling at Rate of $10,000 a Year," *Courier-Journal*, June 2, 1949, 17; Louisville and Jefferson County Board of Health, monthly progress reports, July 1949, February 1952, April 1954; Louisville and Jefferson County Board of Health, meeting minutes, June 28, 1956; "Board of Health Workers Get 8 Per Cent Pay Increase," *Courier-Journal*, March 21, 1952, 27.

142. Louisville and Jefferson County Board of Health, monthly progress reports, October 1949, November 1950, August 1951, July 1953, August 1953, 1947 annual report, 75; "3 City and County Institutions' Farms Rake in Crops and Cash Surpluses," *Courier-Journal*, August 8, 1948, 12.

143. Louisville and Jefferson County Board of Health, annual report, 1946, 94–95.

144. "Barker Urges State Support of Waverly," *Courier-Journal*, January 17, 1948, 9; "Small Budget and Heavier Duties Face Health Board," *Courier-Journal*, April 8, 1950, 7; "The City's Proposed New Budget Is Accompanied by Ominous Signs for '52," *Courier-Journal*, June 17, 1951, 44.

145. Louisville and Jefferson County Board of Health, meeting minutes, June 20, 1946, January 17, 1947; "Health Board Orders Big Cut in Services for Lack of Funds," *Courier-Journal*, June 21, 1946, 1, 9; "What's Rotten in Our City-County Health Budget?," Editorial, *Courier-Journal*, June 22, 1946, 6; "The Good Work of Waverly Hills," *Courier-Journal*, June 26, 1946, 6; "2 Hospitals to Discharge 112 Patients," *Courier Journal*, June

26, 1946, Sec. 2, 15; "Hospital Facilities Cut, Patients Sent Away as City, County Fail to Provide Enough Funds," *Courier-Journal*, June 30, 1946, Sec. 3, 1; Louisville and Jefferson County Board of Health, annual report, 1946, 83.

146. Louisville and Jefferson County Board of Health, meeting minutes, July 26, 1946; "Waverly to Charge Those Able to Pay," *Courier-Journal*, July 27, 1946, 1.

147. "65 Discharged at General Because of Low Funds," *Courier-Journal*, July 31, 1946, 9; Daniel Sledge, *Health Divided: Public Health and Individual Medicine in the Making of the Modern American State* (Lawrence: University Press of Kansas, 2017).

148. "Wants Waverly Free for All," The Point of View, *Courier-Journal*, August 2, 1946, 6.

149. "50 Waverly Hill Patients Able to Make Payments," *Courier-Journal*, October 3, 1946, 20; Louisville and Jefferson County Board of Health, meeting minutes, July 26, 1946, October 18, 1946.

150. Louisville and Jefferson County Board of Health, meeting minutes, December 20, 1950; "Some Patients Able to Pay at Waverly Won't Do So," *Courier-Journal*, December 21, 1950, 65; "Public Hospitals Try to Collect," *Courier-Journal*, January 5, 1951, 6; "35 to 40 Pct. of General's Patients Falsify Ability to Pay," *Courier-Journal*, May 18, 1956, 26.

151. "Some Patients Able to Pay at Waverly Won't Do So," *Courier-Journal*, December 21, 1950, 65; Louisville and Jefferson County Board of Health, monthly progress report, February 1951.

152. "Brock Resigns as Medical Chief at Waverly Hills; Takes a V.A. Post," *Courier-Journal*, February 23, 1946, 3; "History of Waverly Hills Sanatorium," 6; Louisville and Jefferson County Board of Health, 1946 annual report, 81, meeting minutes, September 16, 1943, May 10, 1945, November 1, 1956; "Cooper Brougher to Head Labs at General Hospital," *Courier-Journal*, September 16, 1949, 35; "Latvian Doctor on Waverly Staff Hesitates to Say Too Much of Russia," *Courier-Journal*, November 13, 1949, 14; "They Celebrate Our Way," *Courier-Journal*, November 27, 1949, 64.

153. Louisville and Jefferson County Board of Health, meeting minutes, December 13, 1946, 1947 annual report, 63; "Hospital-Kitchen Bids to Be Asked by Health Board," *Courier-Journal*, December 14, 1946, 9; "Waverly Hills to Help Train Negro Doctors," *Courier-Journal*, April 5, 1947, 9; "We Plan to Study the Negro's Status," *Courier-Journal*, April 13, 1940, 6; Kerns, *Survey of the Economic and Cultural Conditions of the Negro Population of Louisville*, 81–82; "2 Negro Doctors Here Are Appointed to Faculty of U of L Medical School," *Courier-Journal*, December 17, 1953, 21.

154. Louisville and Jefferson County Board of Health, 1947 annual report, 63; "Nurse's Death 7th of Year on Dixie," *Courier-Journal*, May 26, 1954, 11; "Waverly Hills Nursing Chief Is Dead at 66," *Courier-Journal*, August 15, 1954, 25; "Former Waverly Employee Held in Illegal-Liquor Case," *Courier-Journal*, October 9, 1954, 11.
155. "Waverly Hills Orderly Held for Killing Another," *Courier-Journal*, March 2, 1954, 15; "Waverly Hills Orderly Acquitted of Murder in Co-workers' Death," *Courier-Journal*, April 22, 1954, 25; J. Frank W. Stewart, MD, *Sunrise, Sunset: An Autobiography* (New York: Vantage Press, 1991), 100.
156. "New Quarters Held Needed at Waverly," *Courier-Journal*, January 26, 1954, 15; Louisville and Jefferson County Board of Health, meeting minutes, March 1, September 2, September 23, October 22, 1954; July 13, 1955; "Health Unit Wants to Halt Examining First Graders," *Courier-Journal*, September 3, 1954; "Negro Employees' Quarters at Sanatorium Called 'Impossible,'" *Courier-Journal*, January 24, 1957, 15.
157. Louisville and Jefferson County Board of Health, meeting minutes, January 1958; "Sanatorium Reaps Big Dividends on Renovated Workers' Quarters," *Courier-Journal*, November 23, 1958, 23.
158. Louisville and Jefferson County Board of Health, meeting minutes, October 16, 1958; "Sanatorium Reaps Big Dividends on Renovated Workers' Quarters," *Courier-Journal*, November 23, 1958, 23.

Chapter 7

159. Louisville and Jefferson County Board of Health, 1953–54 annual report, 18.
160. Fanelli, "Study of Forty-Three Patients Who Left Waverly Hills," 28; Louisville and Jefferson County Board of Health, 1947 annual report, 86, 74.
161. Fanelli, "Study of Forty-Three Patients Who Left Waverly Hills," 6–7, 26.
162. Ibid., 16, 20.
163. Ibid., 18–19.
164. Ibid., 16, 21, 57.
165. "Waverly Hills Gets New Social Worker," *Courier-Journal*, April 6, 1945, 24; "Social Worker Aids T.B. Patients," *Courier-Journal*, December 22, 1950, 21.
166. Louisville and Jefferson County Health Department, 1944 annual report, 99.
167. Ibid.; 1945 annual report, 90, 94; 1946 annual report, 82. On the expansion of health services for Black patients within racially segregated programs and hospitals, see Karen Kruse Thomas, *Deluxe Jim Crow: Civil*

Rights and American Health Policy, 1935–1954 (Athens: University of Georgia Press, 2011).

168. Louisville and Jefferson County Board of Health, 1946 annual report, 87.

169. Louisville and Jefferson County Health Department, 1944 annual report, 96–97; "Waverly Hills Patients Learn as They Mend," *Courier-Journal*, December 25, 1945, 1; "Silvercrest Starts Off a Rehabilitation Program," *Courier-Journal*, December 2, 1951, 168; "T.B. Victim Gets Help from Christmas Seals," *Courier-Journal*, December 13, 1953, 23.

170. "Back to Normal Living," *Courier-Journal*, November 21, 1954, 184.

171. "T.B. Victim Gets Help from Christmas Seals," *Courier-Journal*, December 13, 1953, 23.

172. "Indebted to Christmas Seals," *Courier-Journal*, December 18, 1953, 8.

173. "New Rehab Center at Waverly Is a Homemaker's Dream," *Courier-Journal*, April 18, 1957, 14.

174. "Doctors Give Waverly Hills Clean Bill," *Courier-Journal*, December 21, 1945, 1, 16.

175. Notes from telephone conversation of Tom Owen with Jeri Gordon Brown, September 5, 2001, reference file on Health: Waverly Hills.

176. Letter from Pauline King to Tom Owen, received October 2, 2002, reference file on Health: Waverly Hills.

177. "New Group Focuses on TB Hospital," *Courier-Journal*, September 25, 2002, clipping in reference file on Health: Waverly Hills.

178. "Church Choir and Family Help Youth at Waverly Hills Mark 17," *Courier-Journal*, August 1, 1955, 12.

179. Stewart, *Sunrise, Sunset*, 105.

180. "Phair Discusses Plan to Shorten Patients' Stay at Waverly Hills," *Courier-Journal*, August 21, 1946, 17; Bynum, *Spitting Blood*, 180.

181. Phone call with Dr. Morris Weiss Jr., May 10, 2021; Louisville and Jefferson County Board of Health, 1944 annual report, meeting minutes, November 29, 1945; 1946 annual report, 29, 82–83; 1947 annual report, 63.

182. Louisville and Jefferson County Board of Health, 1946 annual report, 84; 1947 annual report, 62; meeting minutes, January 17, 1947; Exhibit 7: Letter from Alvin B. Mullen to Dr. John J. Phair, Director of Health, January 10, 1947; meeting minutes, June 20, 1947; "Tuberculosis Death Rate Here Hits New Low but Still Tops U.S. Mark," *Courier-Journal*, January 18, 1948, 10; "New Drug Is Being Used at Waverly and Hazelwood," *Courier-Journal*, December 7, 1948, 15.

183. "3 Hospitals in Area Testing New T.B. Drugs," *Courier-Journal*, May 9, 1952, 36; "New Drugs Aiding Fight Against T.B. in Four Hospitals in the Louisville Area," *Courier-Journal*, August 3, 1952, 27; "Some Ailments of Babies Need Early Surgery," *Courier-Journal*, September 26, 1953, 4; "365

Patients Is Average at Waverly," *Courier-Journal*, December 4, 1955, 17; Bynum, *Spitting Blood*, 190–216.

184. Louisville and Jefferson County Board of Health, 1946 annual report, 84; 1947 annual report, 62.

185. "Waverly Hills Gets Top Rating from Surgeons," *Courier-Journal*, November 14, 1948, 14; Louisville and Jefferson County Board of Health, monthly progress reports, January and February 1949, May and June 1953; letter from Malcolm T. MacEachern, MD, to Mr. Ruskjer, November 3, 1948, Waverly Hills Sanatorium…Proposed Items of Capital Expenditures, Fiscal Year, 1948–1949, meeting minutes, January 16, 1953, November 24, 1954; By-Laws of the Medical Staff of Waverly Hills Sanatorium, January 23, 1956.

186. Louisville and Jefferson County Board of Health, 1953–54 annual report, 18; 1954–55 annual report, 19; 1955–56 annual report, 39; "365 Patients Is Average at Waverly," *Courier-Journal*, December 4, 1955, 17.

187. "Some T.B. Cases Allowed to Leave Waverly Hills, Continue as Outpatients," *Courier-Journal*, February 17, 1956, 3; Louisville and Jefferson County Board of Health, 1956–57 annual report.

188. Steve Russell Video Productions, *Living on the Porch: The Margaret Baugh Waverly Hills Interview*, www.youtube.com/watch?v=AP5JzwdbFiI.

189. "City Hits High Tobacco Spot," *Courier-Journal*, January 1, 1950, 13; meeting with Evelyn Knight Helm at the Filson Historical Society, June 10, 2019.

190. Evelyn Knight Helm autograph book, 1950–51, Mss. C H, FHS.

Chapter 8

191. "From Paris to Glasgow: The Razed TB State Hospitals of Kentucky," tuberculararchitectureofthesouth.wordpress.com/2016/02/04/from-paris-to-glasgow-the-razed-tb-state-hospitals-of-kentucky; *Courier-Journal*, January 16, 1952, 1, 12.

192. Louisville and Jefferson County Board of Health, 1954–55 annual report, 19; "Law May Force T.B. Patient Here into Sanatorium," *Courier-Journal*, May 10, 1955, 17; "Waverly Hills Doing Good Job with TB, Medical Men Agree," *Courier-Journal*, December 11, 1955, sec. 3, 1. Kentucky Revised Statute 214-350 was enacted in 1954 and repealed in 1970: apps.legislature.ky.gov/law/statutes/chapter.aspx?id=38211.

193. "Law May Force T.B. Patient Here into Sanatorium," *Courier-Journal*, May 10, 1955, 17; "Court Orders Father of Seven to T.B. Hospital for 6 Months," *Courier-Journal*, May 11, 1955, 14.

194. "Waverly Hills Doing Good Job with TB, Medical Men Agree," *Courier-Journal*, December 11, 1955, 83.

195. "Report Seeks to Solve Problem of Patients' Leaving Hospitals Uncured," *Courier-Journal*, May 1, 1958, 17; "People Who Won't Finish Treatment Help Keep State TB Rate Near Top," *Courier-Journal*, June 8, 1958, 76.
196. "Why the Hubbub about TB?," *Courier-Journal*, October 25, 1959, 64; "Doctors Say T.B. Care State's Job," *Courier-Journal*, September 13, 1959, 1, 12.
197. "Health, T.B. Groups Discuss Merger or the Operation of Waverly Hills," *Courier-Journal*, September 5, 1959, 9; "Waverly Hills Shift Terms Are Discussed," *Courier-Journal*, July 18, 1959, 1, 12; "State Defers Stand on Waverly Hills," *Courier-Journal*, July 22, 1959; "Physician Challenges Any Move to Close or Limit Waverly Hills," *Courier-Journal*, October 21, 1959, 1, 18; Louisville and Jefferson County Board of Health, meeting minutes, January 28, 1960; "Why the Hubbub about TB?," *Courier-Journal*, October 25, 1959, 64.
198. "T.B. Being Conquered, State Official Declares," *Courier-Journal*, November 24, 1959, 4.
199. "Combs to Urge Closing Waverly Hills Next Year," *Courier-Journal*, January 21, 1960, 1.
200. "Readers' Point of View," *Courier-Journal*, March 20, February 2, February 12, 1960.
201. "Readers' Point of View," *Courier-Journal*, February 13, 1960, 6.
202. "Many Questions about Waverly," *Courier-Journal*, December 6, 1955, 8.
203. "For Moving Sanatorium," *Courier-Journal*, September 20, 1959, 69.
204. "Waverly Hills Wants to Stay Useful," *Courier-Journal*, November 24, 1960, 4.
205. "Mayor Wants Waverly Hills to Help Pay for Community Health Work," *Courier-Journal*, July 24, 1960, 63; "State May Take Over Waverly Sanatorium," *Courier-Journal*, January 12, 1961, 1.
206. "Offer to Lease Waverly Hills for Nursing Home Is Made," *Courier-Journal*, September 30, 1960, 12; Louisville and Jefferson County Board of Health, hearing, September 29, 1960; "Waverly Hills Sanatorium: Should It Be Mentally Retarded Hospital or Park?," *Courier-Journal*, September 17, 1961, 28; "County Approves Plans for Waverly Hills Park," *Courier-Journal*, July 18, 1963, 17; "Park Dollars May Increase," *Courier-Journal*, July 5, 1965, 37.
207. Louisville and Jefferson County Board of Health, meeting minutes, June 23, 1960.
208. "Hazelwood's Andrew Jackson Spry, Talkative at 105—Or 106," *Courier-Journal*, December 4, 1960, 40.

209. S.A. Ruskjer, administrator, to John B. Buschemeyer, September 2, 1960, Box 14, Louisville General Hospital/University Hospital Administrative Office Records, 1991-079, ULASC.
210. Louisville and Jefferson County Board of Health, meeting minutes, October 27, 1960, February 23, 1961, Waverly Hills Sanatorium medical report, October 1960.
211. Louisville and Jefferson County Board of Health, meeting minutes, July 28, 1960; "Hazelwood Costs Hit $785,000," *Courier-Journal*, July 15, 1960, 17; "Patients Juggled as Hazelwood Is Being Improved," *Courier-Journal*, April 9, 1961, 25; "State's Strides Hailed in Fight against T.B.," *Courier-Journal*, October 18, 1961, 17.
212. Louisville and Jefferson County Board of Health, meeting minutes, August 25, 1960; February 23, 1961; "Waverly Hills: End and Beginning," *Courier-Journal*, June 2, 1961, 6.
213. "Waverly Hills Head to Be a Consultant," *Courier-Journal*, June 24, 1961, 4; Louisville and Jefferson County Board of Health, meeting minutes, October 26, 1961; "Hospital Ground Names Ex-Head of Waverly Hills," *Courier-Journal*, September 28, 1961, 12; "Ruskjer Dies of Heart Attack," *Courier-Journal*, November 24, 1961, 17.
214. Louisville and Jefferson County Board of Health, meeting minutes, June 22, 1961; John B. Buschemeyer, director, to Kentucky Security Police, June 12, 1962, Box 14, Louisville General Hospital/University Hospital Administrative Office Records.
215. "Releases to be made up for following employees at Waverly Hills Sanatorium as of June 30, 1962—Job Abolished," Box 14, Louisville General Hospital/University Hospital Administrative Office Records.
216. "Readers' Point of View," *Courier-Journal*, June 8, 1961, 10.

Chapter 9

217. "Lease Signing Launches Center for the Aged at Waverly Hills," *Courier-Journal*, October 17, 1962, 17; "Woodhaven Medical Services: A New Name and a New Role," *Courier-Journal*, April 11, 1970, 6; "Home's Plan to Close Ends State's Most Intense Probe," *Courier-Journal*, December 15, 1980, 6; "Last 10 Patients Leave Criticized Nursing Home," *Courier-Journal*, January 1, 1981, 1; email from Emma Johansen, December 1, 2021.
218. "Historic Hospital Could Be Torn Down," *Courier-Journal*, March 10, 2001, clipping in reference file on Health: Waverly Hills.
219. City of Louisville, *Annual Reports for the Fiscal Year Ending August 31, 1916 and December 31, 1916* (Louisville, KY: Geo. G. Fetter Company), 427;

Louisville and Jefferson County Health Department, 1959–60 statistical report, 60.

220. For references to treatments and surgeries at Waverly Hills as "barbaric" and "experimental," see "Waverly Hills: Once Famed for 'White Plague' Treatment, Old Hospital Has Become a White Elephant," *Courier-Journal*, August 13–14, 8; "Waverly Hills Sanatorium Still Source of Local Curiosity," *Cardinal*, October 21, 2003; "The Death Tunnel," *Courier-Journal*, May 15, 2004, 14, clippings in reference file on Health: Waverly Hills.

221. For examples of claims of fifty thousand to sixty-four thousand total deaths, or a patient every hour dying in the first few years of the sanatorium, see "The Haunted Hospital," www.mentalfloss.com/article/17263/haunted-hospital; "The Unconventional Convention: Louisville Plays Host to Mid-South Paranormal Convention," *Leo Weekly*, September 18, 2002, 6–7, clipping in reference file on Health: Waverly Hills; "Waverly Hills Sanatorium Continues Reconstruction," *Cardinal*, October 26, 2004, clipping in reference file on Health: Waverly Hills; "The Legend of Louisville's Haunted Hospital: Waverly Hills Sanatorium," www.wlky.com/article/the-legend-of-louisville-s-spooky-waverly-hills-sanatorium/38090750.

222. Emerson and Phillips, *Hospitals and Health Agencies of Louisville 1924*, 44, 48–49, 52.

223. John and Angela Amerine spreadsheets, shared with author. See also Kentucky Historic Institutions, "WHS: Patient Death Index," kyhi.org/waverly-hills-patient-death-index.

224. Louisville and Jefferson County Health Department, 1944 annual report, 100–1.

225. *Louisville Leader*, August 18, 1923, October 20, 1928, February 28, 1931; 1930 United States federal census, ancestry.com.

226. Obituaries, *Courier-Journal*, October 13, 1926, 5; "William B. Harold, 66, Commits Suicide at Home," *Courier-Journal*, August 5, 1921, 8.

227. Stewart, *Sunrise, Sunset*, 99.

228. "Waverly Hills: Once Famed for 'White Plague' Treatment, Old Hospital Has Become a White Elephant." See also "Waverly Hills," *Courier-Journal*, November 23, 1989, 102.

229. "$1,000,000 for Hospital Urged," *Courier-Journal*, January 1, 1922, 5; *Living on the Porch*.

230. "Body Consigned to Pickling Vat Is Recovered by Dead Man's Relatives," *Courier-Journal*, August 28, 1912, 8.

231. Louisville and Jefferson County Board of Health, meeting minutes, May 19, 1955.

232. "Hospital's Corrective Measures Are Praised," *Courier-Journal*, May 20, 1955, 39.

233. Edward C. Halperin, "The Poor, the Black, and the Marginalized as the Source of Cadavers in United States Anatomical Education," *Clinical Anatomy* 20 (2007): 489–95; "Corpses, Body-Cutting Instruments Can Be Found in Medical School Laboratory," *Cardinal*, April 9, 1936, 4; "Medics Had to Dig up Lab Material in the 80s," *Courier-Journal Sunday Magazine*, May 19, 1940; Ky. Rev. Statute 311.330, Recodified 1942 Ky. Acts ch. 208, sec. 1, effective October 1, 1942, from Ky. Stat. sec. 2647.

234. World Health Organization, "Tuberculosis," www.who.int/newsroom/fact-sheets/detail/tuberculosis.

ABOUT THE AUTHOR

Lynn Pohl holds a BS in history from Millsaps College in Jackson, Mississippi, and an MA and PhD in history from Indiana University–Bloomington. She has taught history at Indiana University and at colleges in Asheville, North Carolina, and Louisville, Kentucky. She moved with her family to Louisville in 2006 to live in the same neighborhood as her sister, and she hopes to remain in her adopted hometown for many more years. She has worked at the Filson Historical Society since 2018.